# THE
# POWERBAND
## WORKOUT

# THE POWER

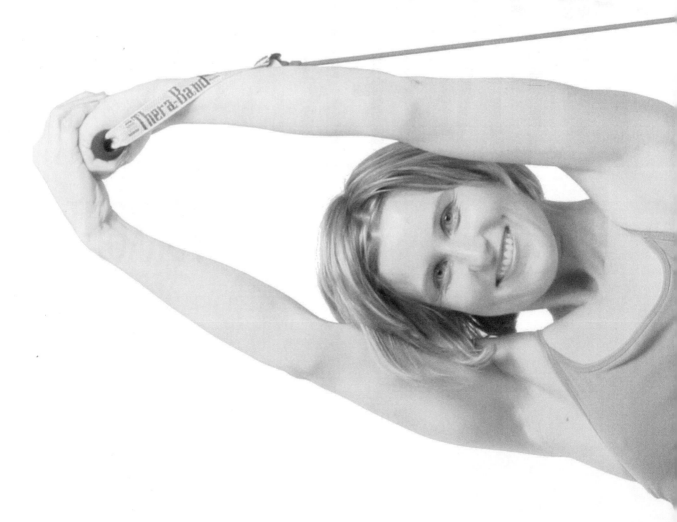

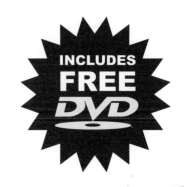
**INCLUDES FREE DVD**

# BAND WORKOUT

## The Easiest Way to Shape and Sculpt— All You Need Is Your Body and the Band

### *By* PAUL FREDIANI

PHOTOGRAPHS
*by* PETER FIELD PECK

**healthy**living**books**
NEW YORK · LONDON

Published by Hatherleigh Press
5-22 46th Avenue, Suite 200
Long Island City, NY 11101
Visit our Web site:
www.healthylivingbooks.com

Library of Congress Cataloging-in-Publication Data

Frediani, Paul, 1952-
    The powerband workout : the easiest way to shape and sculpt—all you need is your body and the band / by Paul Frediani ; photographs by Peter Field Peck.
        p. cm.
    "Includes Free DVD."
    ISBN 1-57826-200-3
    1.  Exercise--Miscellanea. 2.  Physical fitness--Miscellanea.  I. Title.
    RA781.F74 2005
    613.7'10284--dc22

Seek the advice of your physician before starting any physical fitness program.

HEALTHY LIVING BOOKS are available for bulk purchase, special promotions, and premiums. For information on reselling and special purchase opportunities, please call us at 1-800-528-2550 and ask for the Special Sales Manager.

Cover and interior design by Corin Hirsch and Deborah Miller

Special thanks to Mark Anderson and Naomi Kall at The Hygenic Corporation for the use of Thera-Band equipment featured in the photos.

10 9 8 7 6 5 4 3 2 1
Printed in the United States

# *Acknowledgments*

Special thanks to my publisher Andrew Flach, my editor Andrea Au, art director/production manager Deborah Miller, assistant editor Alyssa Smith, photographer Peter Peck, and our models, Andrea Sooch and Rebecca Houck. All made working on *The PowerBand Workout* a pleasure. I'd also like to thank the educators in the fitness industry that have elevated the level and knowledge of fitness professionals. Special thanks to Paul Chek and Juan Carlos Santana for their inspiring workshops and seminars.

To my clients for their support and trust.

Most of all, thank you to my family and friends who have always believed in me.

# Table of
# Conte

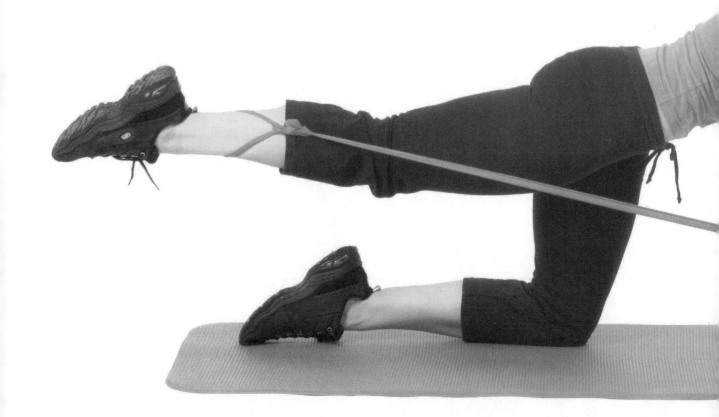

nts

### Chapter 1

# Welcome
## *to* PowerBand

The Rolling Stones said, "Time is on my side." We all know that's not life in the 21st century. From the moment we wake up in the morning until we go to bed in the night, the clock is ticking, and trying to get everything done sometimes seems impossible.

The last thing on our minds is fitting one more thing into our already crowded schedules. Who has the luxury of one to two hours to exercise?

Everyone knows how important exercise is. A day doesn't go by when its importance is not highlighted. Exercising is without a doubt the single most important thing you can do to improve your health and longevity. There is no magic pill; we must include exercise in our everyday life as routinely as we brush our teeth.

But even if you find the time to exercise, there are so many questions you will have. Just where do you start? Will you need to know anything about exercise machines or equipment? Can

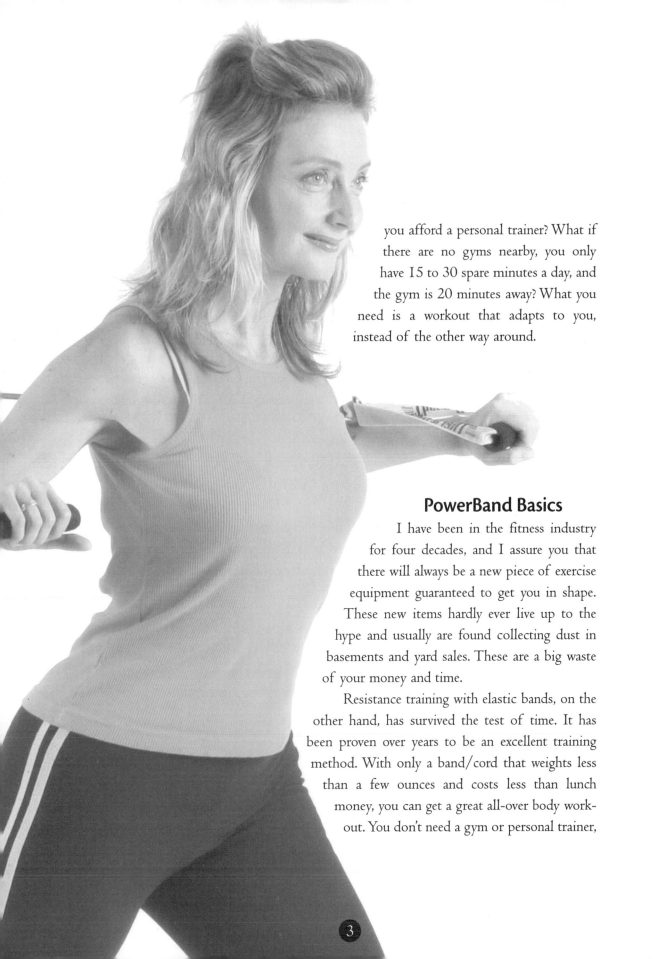

you afford a personal trainer? What if there are no gyms nearby, you only have 15 to 30 spare minutes a day, and the gym is 20 minutes away? What you need is a workout that adapts to you, instead of the other way around.

## PowerBand Basics

I have been in the fitness industry for four decades, and I assure you that there will always be a new piece of exercise equipment guaranteed to get you in shape. These new items hardly ever live up to the hype and usually are found collecting dust in basements and yard sales. These are a big waste of your money and time.

Resistance training with elastic bands, on the other hand, has survived the test of time. It has been proven over years to be an excellent training method. With only a band/cord that weights less than a few ounces and costs less than lunch money, you can get a great all-over body workout. You don't need a gym or personal trainer,

**CHANGE IS GOOD**
If you never change your exercise routine, you'll never change your body. That's because over time your body adapts to the same routine. If you want to become stronger and more fit, then you must constantly change your workouts. Changing the speed, intensity, and power of an exercise will do just that.

and you can exercise in the privacy of your own home or office. The best thing about the simplicity of the PowerBand workout is that you don't need to be a gym rat in order to follow the program correctly.

The PowerBand Workout was designed to work equally well for beginners and experienced athletes. I have trained athletes of all ages, up to 87 years young, with elastic resistance. The exercises are easily ordered from simple to increasingly challenging.

## Get Ready to Succeed!

The most important qualities in any workout are CDF: Convenient, Doable, and Fun. No exercise program will get results without being CDF. Can you count how many exercise programs you have begun and then given up on? It has been my experience that if an exercise program isn't CDF, then it simply will not hold your attention for long. If you are looking for results, consistency is the key.

Increasing and maintaining strength, endurance, balance, flexibility, and stability are concerns for all of us. Our goal should be to make exercise a part of our everyday lives. I truly believe that there's an athlete hidden inside every one of us, from the mother pushing the shopping cart to the businessman rushing from meeting to meeting. We can do much more than we believe is possible. PowerBand training will bring even more health and energy to your greatest game: Your life.

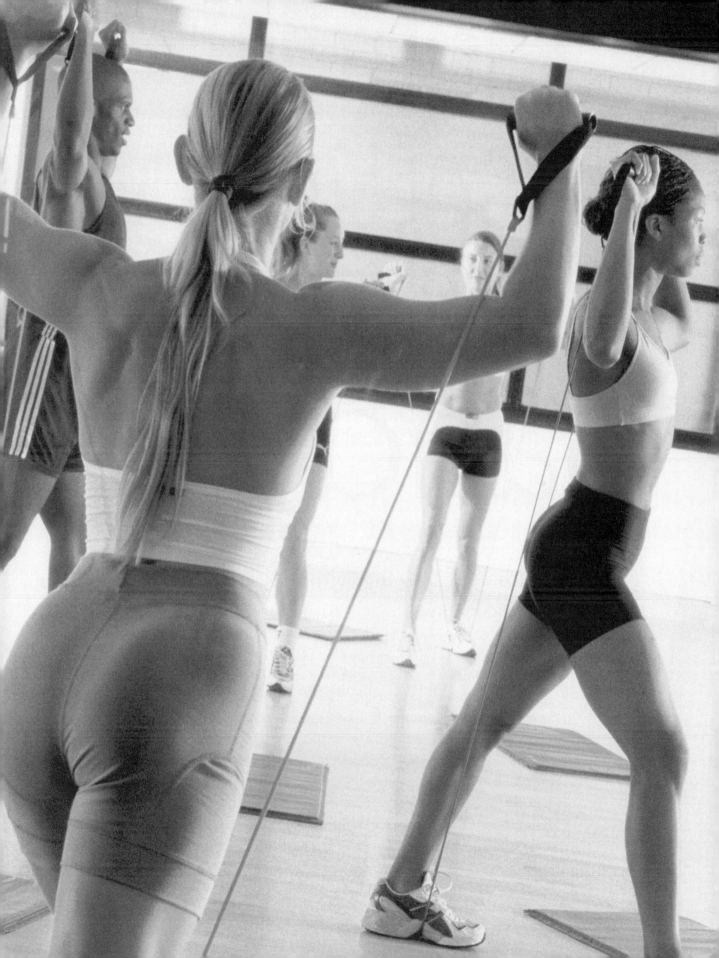

### Chapter 2

# Getting Acquainted *with the* Band

Although training with elastic resistance has been around for many years, it has just recently become a mainstream method of exercising. Used first in physical rehabilitation, it has many other attributes that can contribute to your fitness. There are even things the band can accomplish that other methods of exercise, such as free weights and machines, cannot reproduce.

The band is able to reproduce the body's movements within its natural full range of motion. It can also be part of an effective resistance training workout. It can be used in the most basic exercises or the most advanced, and can adapt to perform at the speed resembling everyday life or the hastened pace found in sports. When we exercise the way we move instead of isolating individual body parts, we develop the whole body, as nature has intended.

Imagine the body you want. You are probably imagining a body that looks natural and esthetically pleasing. Genetics aside, your ideal body is developed by performing exercises that come naturally. Our bodies are built to move fluidly and gracefully, and these movements can be both simple and complex. As children, we learned all of our basic movements,

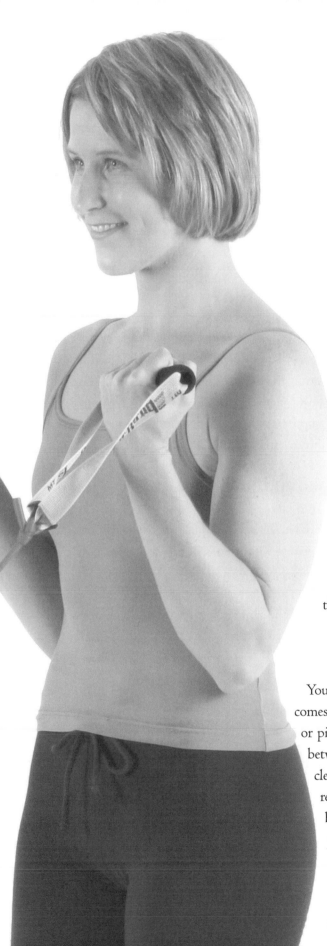

also known as the 4 Pillars of Human Movement (pulling, pushing, pressing, and squatting). The band can assist in developing any of these primary movements.

Exercising with the band is extremely time efficient, and training with it can easily increase your physical conditioning, and improve your strength, flexibility, and performance, as well as reducing your body fat and simplifying your everyday life. Bands also perform just as well for the novice exerciser as they do for the experienced athlete.

## The Science Behind Resistance Training with the Band

Your muscles are blind. They don't know if resistance comes from lifting dumbbells, pushing a shopping cart, or picking up a bag of cement. The greatest difference between the band and free weights is when your muscles receive resistance. Free weights rely on gravity for resistance, while the band does not. Bands, in fact, become more taut the more they are stretched, which increases their resistance.

**POWERBAND TIP**
Pain should never be part of exercise.

If you do experience pain while exercising, stop. Perhaps your posture needs to be reassessed or maybe you're trying to progress too quickly.

Exercising with the band also requires more coordination and stabilization than a machine-based exercise program. When you exercise with the band, it requires you to develop your own pathway of movement, unlike exercise machines, which are on a fixed plane. Exercising without being restricted to one repetitive movement will create a body that is coordinated and moves seamlessly.

By exercising outside a fixed plane, you also activate your stabilizing muscles and core. When you exercise your core, you strengthen the muscles of your abdominals, and also those of your lumbar, thoracic, and cervical spine. Strengthening your smaller stabilizing muscles improves your posture, and strong core stabilizers will allow for improvement of your functional strength. What's the point of being able to bench press 100 pounds on your back if you can't push a 50-pound shopping cart when you're on your feet?

Exercises with the band can be performed at all speeds. Try going controlled and slowly for your general fitness or fast and explosively for your sports performance training. The band also helps your balance when you exercise while standing. For example, if we're standing and moving three-dimensionally, our center of gravity shifts. Balance underlies all our movements and our posture is a crucial part of this. By learning to go outside our base of support and our comfort level, we will improve not only our balance but also our stability, strength, and endurance.

## Band and Tubing Basics

Elastic bands are available in a variety of strengths, which allows you to easily add tension and power to your workout. This, in addition to the many advantages listed above, makes bands uniquely suited to inproving your exercise routine.

You should choose a band with a resistance that allows you to properly execute an exercise with good form. Your first attempts with these exercises will teach your muscles the movement patterns. It's best when first learning not to sacrifice form. As you become experienced with the exercises and can execute them with proper form, increase the resistance of the band or tube. You can further increase the challenge and complexity of an exercise by adding a exercise ball to your routine.

There are very few differences between bands and tubing. Typically, a manufacturer creates bands and tubing of the same resistence level in the same color. (Keep in mind that different manufacturers may use a different color scale.)

For purposes of exercising, there is no difference in the use of a band versus a tube, other than comfort of use. In the PowerBand exercises, we have indicated whether an exercise should be done with a band, a tube, or may be performed with either.

In many exercises, you are asked to anchor your band/tube at a certain point in relation to your height. In addition to using attachments that will allow your workout to take place at a door (the doorknob and top or lower section of a door), there are many other options available to you.

There are some things to be alert to while using a band or tube. Unfortunately, bands and tubing occasionally break. While they are more subject to wear than standard weights, they are, due to testing and many breakthroughs in manufacturing, also extremely durable.

Examine a band right before use, every time, to catch any damage that could cause you to injure yourself. When exercising, make sure the band is securely fastened so it does not snap back unexpectedly.

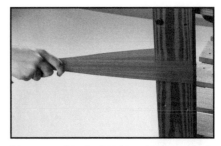
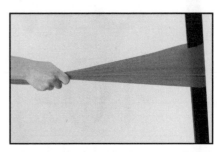
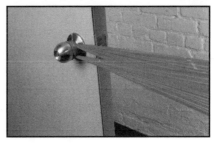

You can anchor the band to a bookcase (top), a pole (middle), or a doorknob (bottom).

## About the PowerBand Workouts

In the pages that follow, you'll learn everything you need to know about working out with exercise bands. You'll start by discovering the many places you can exercise when using the extremely adaptable band. Your home, your office, or even your car turn into a time- and space-saving gym.

After that, you'll move on to the PowerBand 10-Minute Warm-Up. Do these exercises in sequence as a prelude to the more challenging workouts to come.

Chapter 4 is where you'll learn all the PowerBand moves. These exercises will challenge your whole body, strengthening and sculpting your lower and your upper body alike. The band targets eight muscle groups with unique exercises, all clearly illustrated for your use.

In Chapter 5, you will be introduced to exercises specifically designed to enhance your flexibility, using the band's unique properties. Turn the page to Chapter 6 and learn the Big Bang Moves. All of these specially designed exercises work multiple muscle groups at once, cutting your exercise time in half and doubling your workout intensity.

Chapter 7 is where it all comes together in the PowerBand Workout, a progressive six-week body sculpting plan. It couldn't be simpler: One hour a day, three days a week for six weeks. But I don't just throw you a band and wish you luck. My workouts guide you from the very beginning to an advanced body sculpting workout.

So, again, welcome to PowerBand. With the band and this book, I guarantee you a workout like you've never seen!

### Chapter 3

# The PowerBand 10-Minute Warm-Up

Warming up is an essential part of any workout. A 5– to 8–minute warm-up is ideal. Physically, it takes the body a little time to acknowledge that it is about to exercise. If you jump right into exercise without warming up, you not only risk injury, but also will fatigue more quickly and not be as physically efficient. It is also important to put distance between whatever frame of mind you're in and a workout frame of mind. Quite often the first 10 minutes of a workout are not effective because the mind is somewhere else: at work, thinking about a relationship, at the laundry, etc. Give yourself the luxury of the warm-up. It will connect the body and mind and is the best preparation for a great workout.

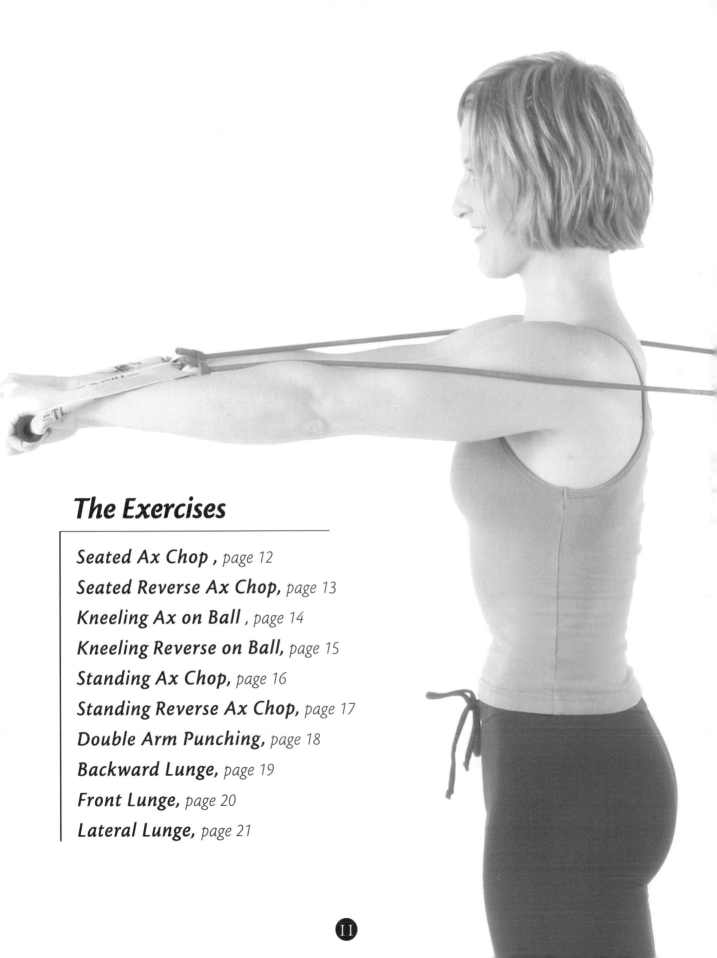

# The Exercises

# Seated Ax Chop

## TECHNIQUE & FORM

Anchor the band overhead. Sit on the apex of the ball, your knees bent at 90 degrees and your feet flat on the floor. Hold the band in your hands and draw the band down from over your shoulder to the opposing hip.

*This exercise can be performed with both the exercise band and tube.*

*Paul's Pro Tip*

The handgrip should always be in the top hand, keeping in mind the direction you are rotating.

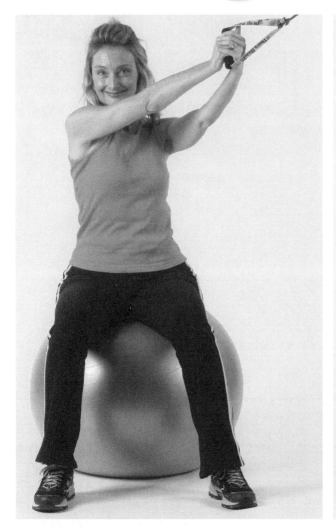
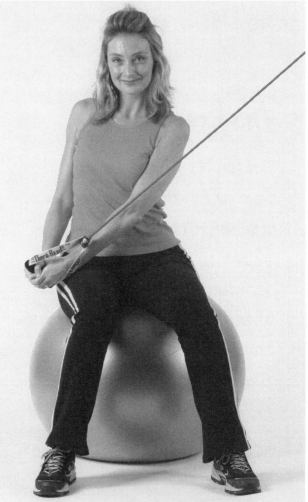

# Seated Reverse Ax Chop

*This exercise can be performed with both the exercise band and tube.*

## TECHNIQUE & FORM

Anchor the band at the floor. Sit on the apex of the ball, knees bent at a 90 degree angle with your feet flat on the floor. Hold the band in your hands. Draw the band up from your hip to the opposite shoulder.

### Paul's Pro Tip

Keep your head and your hips fixed forward. Rotate from the shoulders.

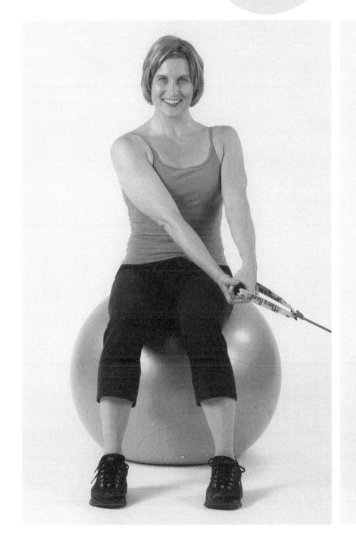
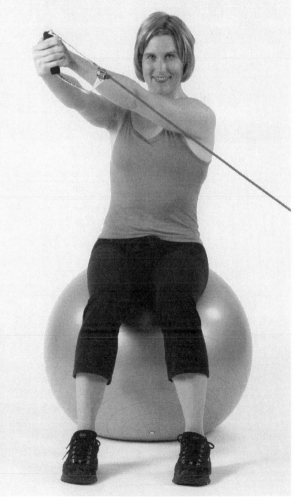

# Kneeling Ax on Ball

*This exercise can be performed with both the exercise band and tube.*

**TECHNIQUE & FORM**

The band should be anchored overhead. With your knees shoulder width apart, kneel on the ball. Hold the band with both hands and draw the band from above your head to the opposite hip.

### Paul's Pro Tip

Kneeling on the ball is an advanced position and this exercise should not be attempted until one is perfectly comfortable kneeling on the ball.

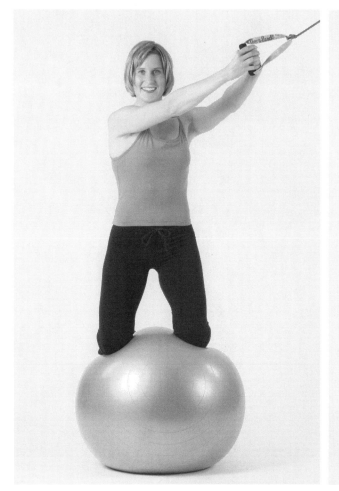
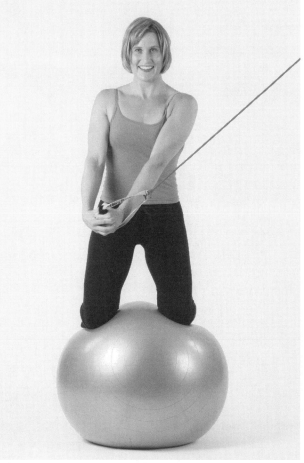

# Kneeling Reverse on Ball

*This exercise can be performed with both the exercise band and tube.*

## Paul's Pro Tip

Drop your butt to your heels and lift your hips up during the upward rotation for a more advanced movement.

## TECHNIQUE & FORM

The band should be anchored to the floor. With your knees shoulder width apart, kneel on the ball. Hold the band with both of your hands and draw the band from your hip to your opposite shoulder.

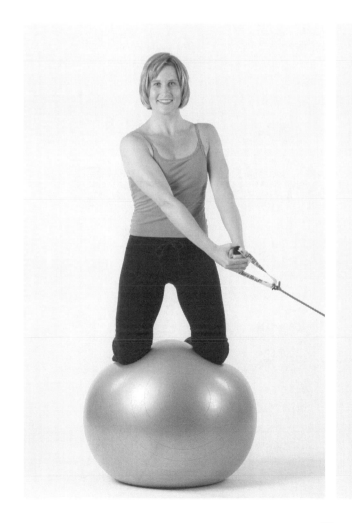

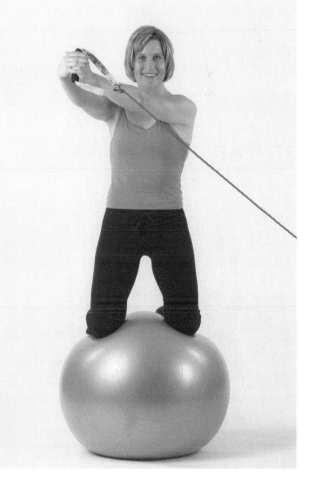

# Standing Ax Chop

## TECHNIQUE & FORM
Anchor the band overhead. Stand with your feet shoulder width apart. Draw the band from over your head to the opposite hip.

*This exercise can be performed with both the exercise band and tube.*

*Paul's Pro Tip*

Keep the natural arch in your back, your abs taut, and your knees slightly bent, and you will relieve any stress in your lower back.

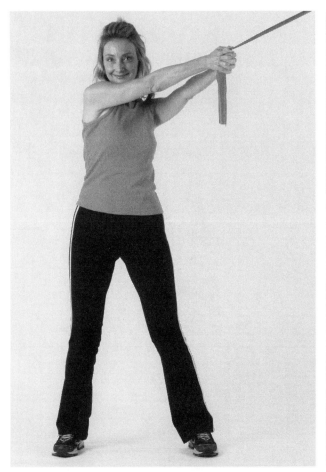
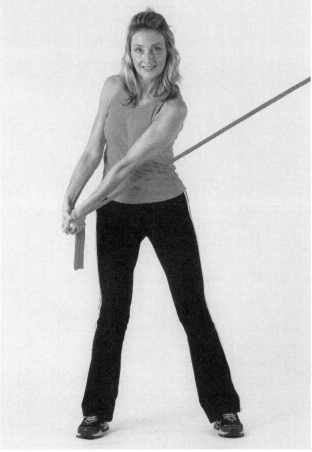

# Standing Reverse Ax Chop

## TECHNIQUE & FORM
Anchor the band to the floor. Stand with your feet shoulder width apart. Draw the band from low at your hip to over the opposite shoulder.

*This exercise can be performed with both the exercise band and tube.*

*Paul's Pro Tip*
Keep your knees slightly bent as you move up from your feet to your hips, trunk, and finally your shoulders.

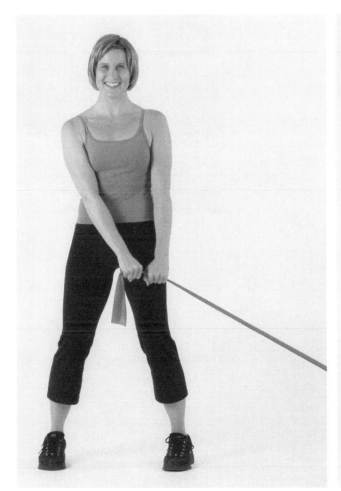

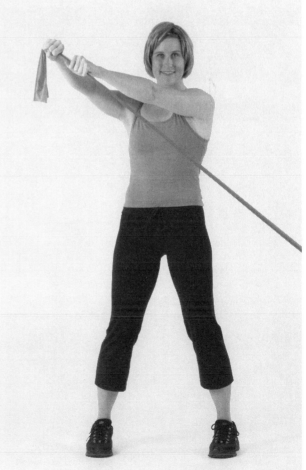

# Double Arm Punching

## TECHNIQUE & FORM

Anchor the band behind you at chest height and hold the band at each end with your hands. Stand in a split lunge position, one foot in front of the other. Alternate punching forward.

*This exercise can be performed with both the exercise band and tube.*

*Paul's Pro Tip*

Be sure the bands are in line with the top of your forearms when arms are extended to avoid shoulder stress. Focus on keeping your shoulder blades back during the entire exercise.

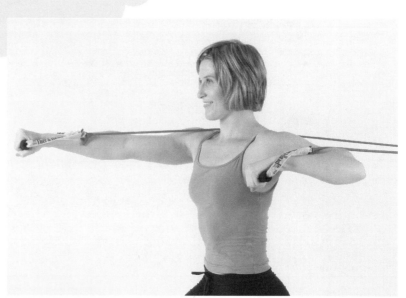

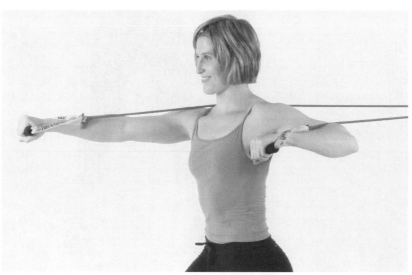

# Backward Lunge

### TECHNIQUE & FORM

Anchor the band at chest height. Stand with your feet hip distance apart. Hold the band at each end. Begin a backward lunge and pull the band back with you simultaneously. Repeat, alternating legs.

*This exercise can be performed with both the exercise band and tube.*

*Paul's Pro Tip*

Avoid leaning forward or backward with your torso during the lunge. Move in a controlled fashion.

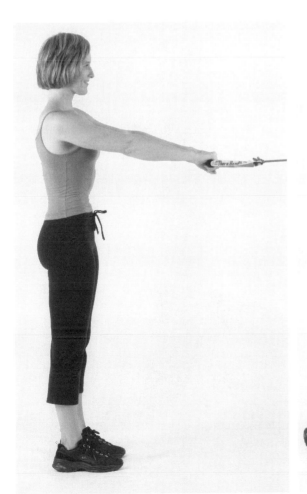

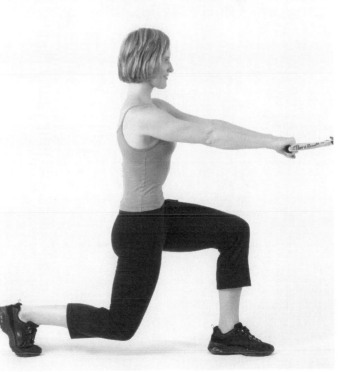

# Front Lunge

*This exercise can be performed with both the exercise band and tube.*

### Paul's Pro Tip
Avoid bouncing the rear knee on the floor. Be sure that your front knee does not extend over your toe. Keep your front knee directly over your ankle while in the lunge position.

## TECHNIQUE & FORM
Anchor the band at chest height. Stand with your feet hip distance apart. Hold the band at each end. Extend your arms in front of your chest and step out in a foward lunge. Repeat, alternating your legs.

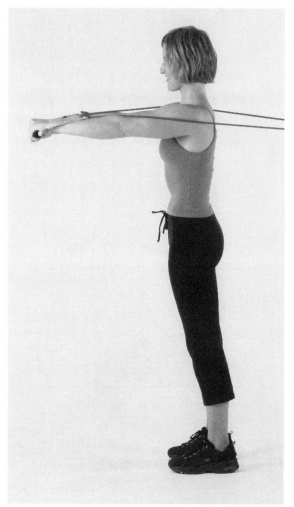
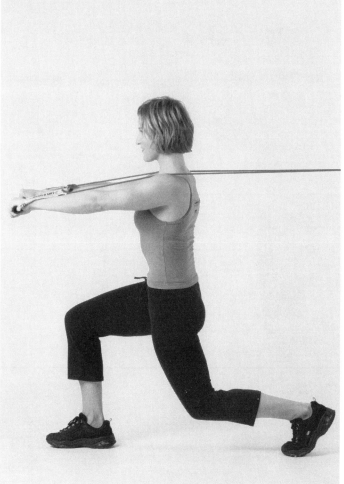

# Lateral Lunge

*This exercise can be performed with both the exercise band and tube.*

### TECHNIQUE & FORM

Anchor the band at waist height. Stand with your feet wider than shoulder width apart. Hold the band with both of your hands at hip height. Holding your arms straight, shift your weight from one leg to the another. Alternate sides.

**Paul's Pro Tip**

Keep your chest high and your shoulders back. Keeping your arms fixed in place will intensify the exercise of your hips and legs.

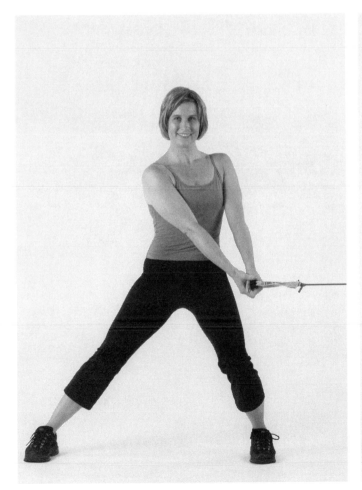
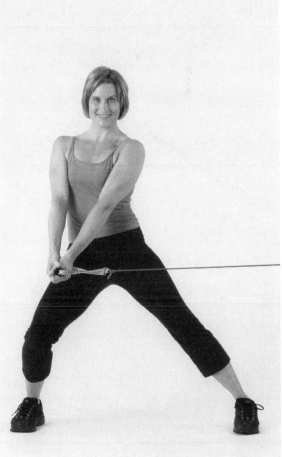

### Chapter 4

# *The* PowerBa

## *Moves*

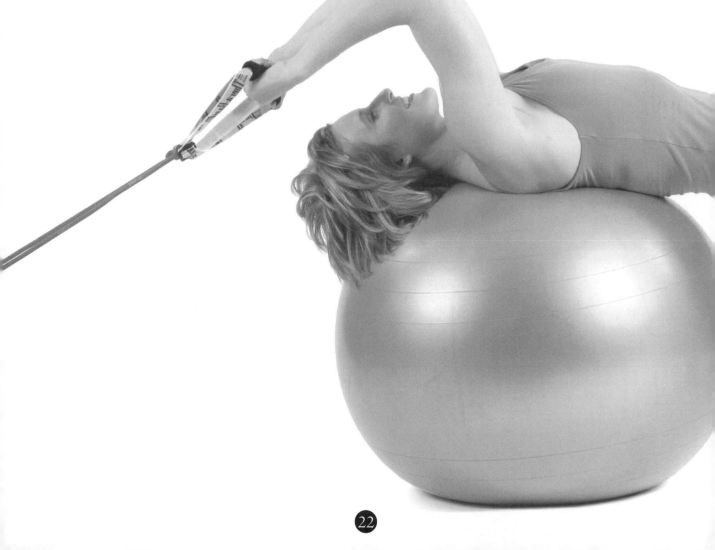

nd

Before beginning the PowerBand Workout, it's always best to do a good warm-up of 5 to 10 minutes. But if time is of the essence, then for the first few minutes of your workout, use bands of very light resistance.

Each of the exercises is designed to target a specific muscle group. However, all of the exercises also require the use of several other muscles in order to execute them smoothly and properly. Several of the exercises will also challenge your balance, developing your core. As a result, you will develop your body as a whole and not in isolated pieces. It's always preferable to perform the exercises in their full range of motion, but always stay within a range that is comfortable to you. You should never force your body into an uncomfortable position. Everyone has a unique body type and its boundaries should be respected. Pain is not gain, but is instead the fast track to injury.

If you have a mirror available, make use of it to monitor your posture. You should never perform an exercise during which you cannot maintain good posture. Finally, you cannot exercise without breathing! Many people make the mistake of holding their breath while exercising. Be sure you breathe naturally and fully during your exercises. This will make your experience more enjoyable and guarantee you better results, injury-free.

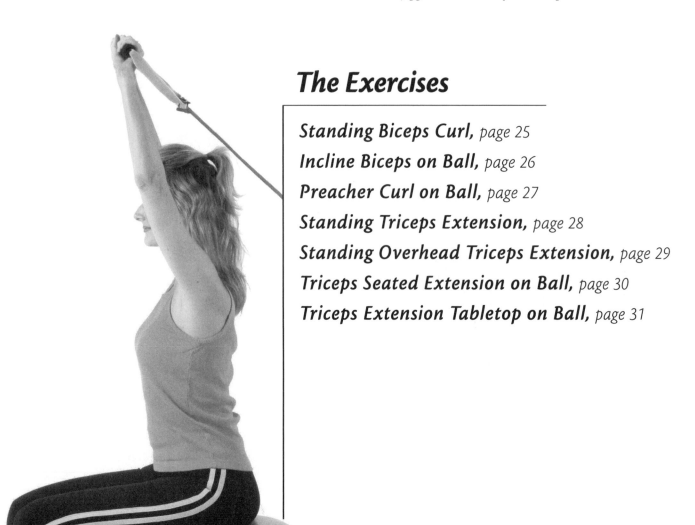

*PowerBand*

# Arms

**Biceps Brachii and Triceps Brachii**

Whether you are in a T-shirt or an evening gown, your arms are going to get attention. Wouldn't you rather have them tight and toned? Target and remove the back-of-the-arm jiggles and define your biceps.

## The Exercises

# Standing Biceps Curl

## TECHNIQUE & FORM

Anchor the band at the floor. Stand with your feet shoulder width apart, keeping your knees slightly bent. Hold each end of the band with hands. Keeping your palms facing forward, draw the band towards your shoulders.

*This exercise can be performed with both the exercise band and tube.*

*Paul's Pro Tip*

Keep your shoulders back and avoid rounding them forward. Keeping your elbows back and against your ribs will give the biceps a greater pump.

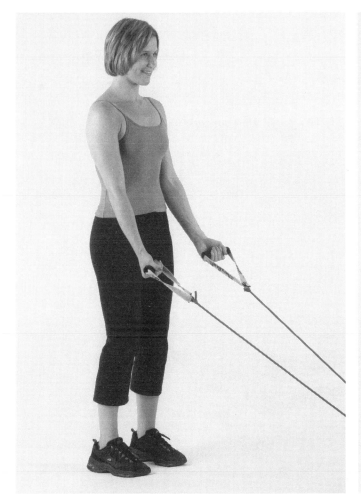
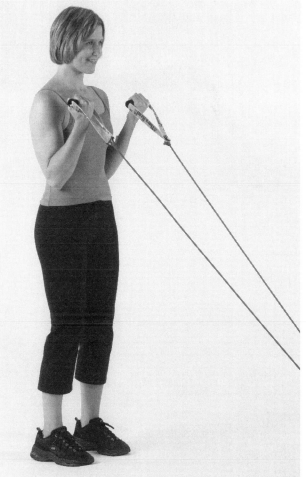

# Incline Biceps on Ball

*This exercise can be performed with both the exercise band and tube.*

### Paul's Pro Tip
Tuck your chin to your chest to help avoid neck stress.

## TECHNIQUE & FORM
Anchor the band at the floor. Sit with your knees bent and your lower back braced against the ball. Lift your hips slightly off the floor. Hold the bands at each end with your palms facing forward. Rest the back of your arms on the ball and draw your hands toward your shoulders.

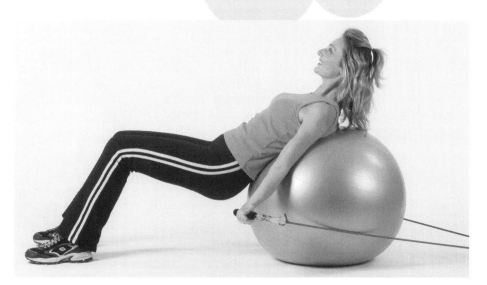

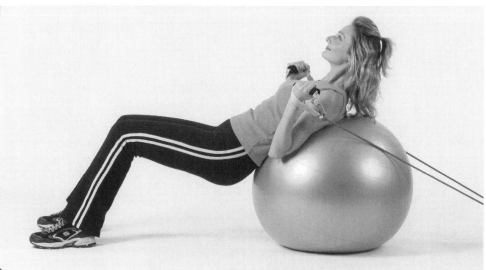

# Preacher Curl on Ball

*This exercise can be performed with both the exercise band and tube.*

### Paul's Pro Tip
Isolating and extending the arm in its fullest range of motion will increase the intensity of this exercise. Try beginning with a light band or resistance.

## TECHNIQUE & FORM
Anchor the band at the floor. Kneel and place your chest and backs of your arms on the ball. Hold band at each end, extending your arms straight ahead. Keep the backs of your arms on the ball and draw your hands toward your shoulders.

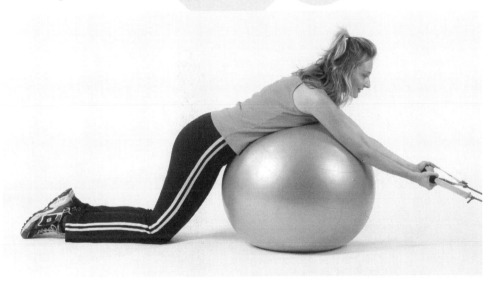

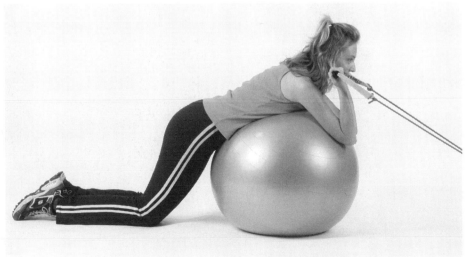

# Standing Triceps Extension

*This exercise can be performed with both the exercise band and tube.*

**TECHNIQUE & FORM**

Anchor the band overhead. Stand with your feet hip distance apart. Hold the band with both hands, with your elbows pressed against your waist and your palms facing the floor. Press your hands down to your hips.

***Paul's Pro Tip***

Be sure to keep your shoulder blades back and press your hands to your hips.

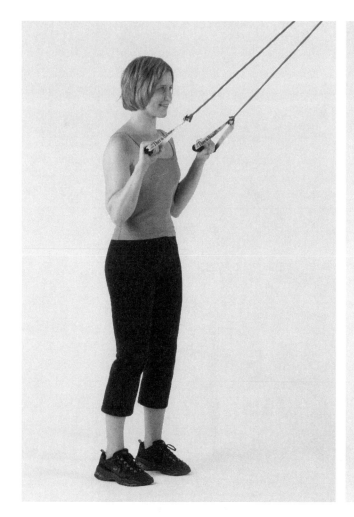

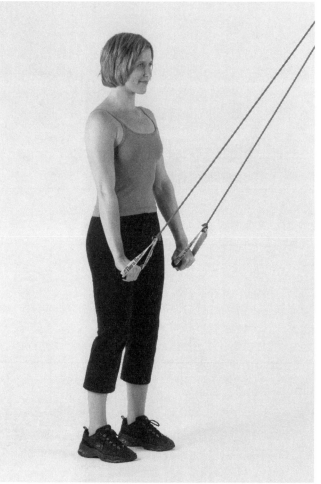

# Standing Overhead Triceps Extension

*This exercise can be performed with both the exercise band and tube.*

### Paul's Pro Tip
Keep your upper arm in a fixed position horizontal to the floor, bending only at the elbow.

## TECHNIQUE & FORM
Anchor the band overhead. Stand in a split leg lunge position, your knees slightly bent. Hold the band with both hands, your palms facing forward and your torso bent slightly forward at the waist. Keep the backs of your arm parallel to the floor. Press your hands forward.

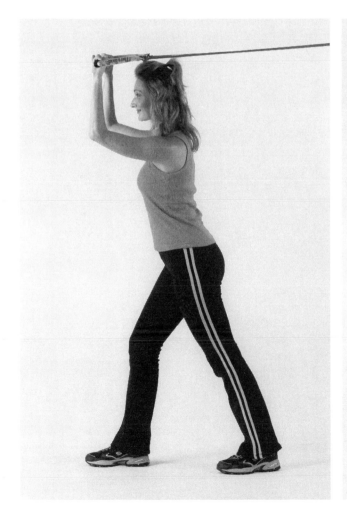
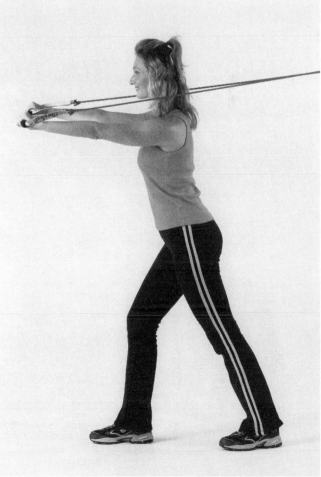

# Triceps Seated
# Extension on Ball

*This exercise can be performed with both the exercise band and tube.*

## TECHNIQUE & FORM

Anchor the band at the floor. Sit on the apex of the ball with your feet flat on the floor. Point your elbows to the ceiling, both of your hands behind your head grasping the band. Press overhead.

*Paul's Pro Tip*

A good way to ease into this push-up is to start by setting the ball against a wall.

## VARIATION

If it's difficult to maintain your balance, place one foot in front of ball and one foot to the side.

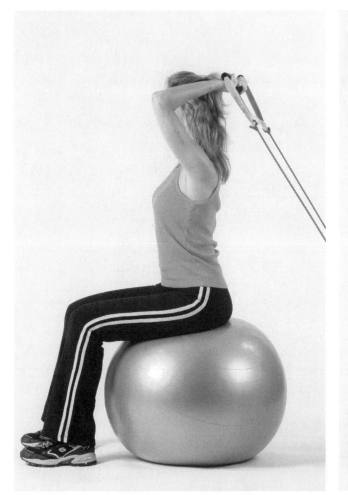 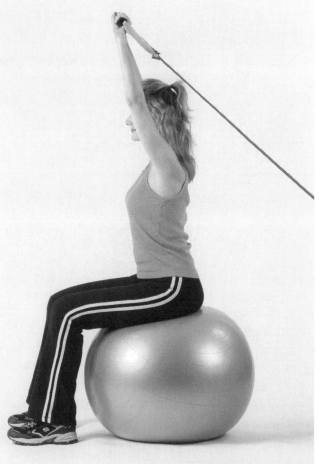

# Triceps Extension
# Tabletop on Ball

*This exercise can be performed with both the exercise band and tube.*

**Paul's Pro Tip**

Keep your knees, hips, and shoulder at same height, parallel to the ground.

## TECHNIQUE & FORM

Anchor the band at the floor. Hold with both hands. Sit on the apex of the ball and roll your body down to a tabletop position. Point your elbows to the ceiling with your arms bent at 90 degrees. Press your arms to a straightened position.

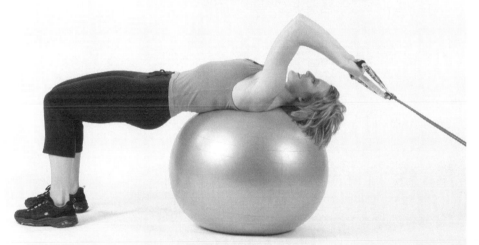

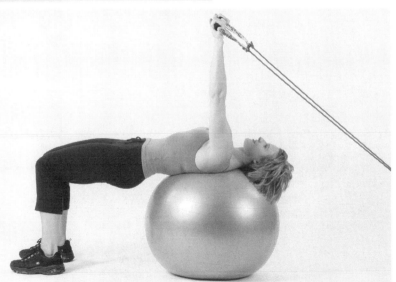

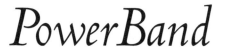

# PowerBand
# Shoulders

**Anterior, Medial, and Posterior Deltoids**

If your goals include sculpted and shapely shoulders, you should definitely indulge in the following exercises. Defined and strong shoulders are not only aesthetic, they keep your upper body injury-free.

## The Exercises

# Shoulder Upright Row

### TECHNIQUE & FORM
Anchor the band at the floor. Stand with your feet shoulder width apart and your knees slightly bent. Hold band with both hands, your palms facing your thighs. Lift your elbow up until the backs of your arms are parallel to your shoulders.

*This exercise can be performed with both the exercise band and tube.*

**Paul's Pro Tip**
Focus on keeping your shoulders down and away from your ears.

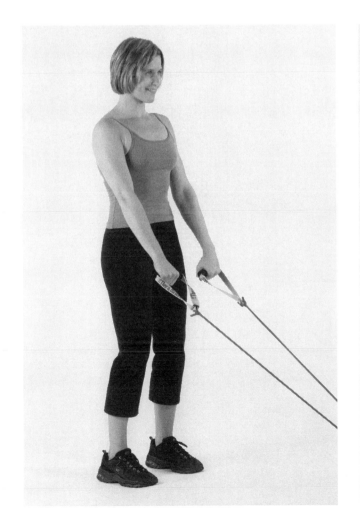
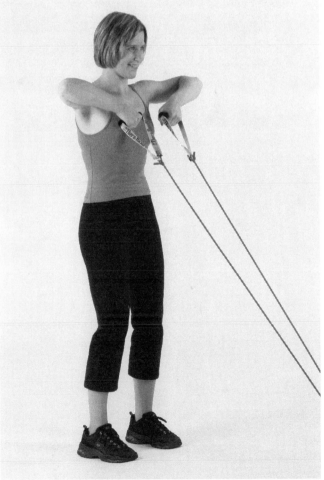

# Shoulder Press

## TECHNIQUE & FORM

Anchor the band to the floor. Stand with your feet shoulder width apart and your knees slightly bent. Hold the band with both of your hands, palms facing the ceiling. Begin with your elbows against your ribs, and then press the bands overhead.

*This exercise can be performed with both the exercise band and tube.*

*Paul's Pro Tip*

Support the lower back by drawing your belly tight before pressing the bands overhead.

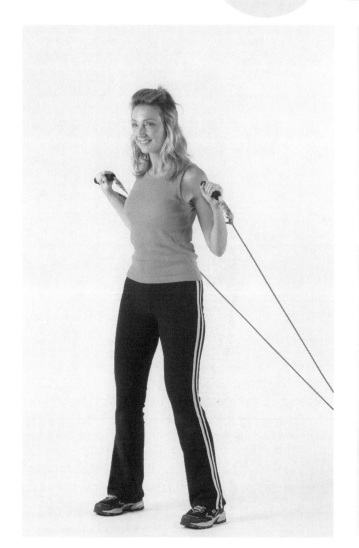
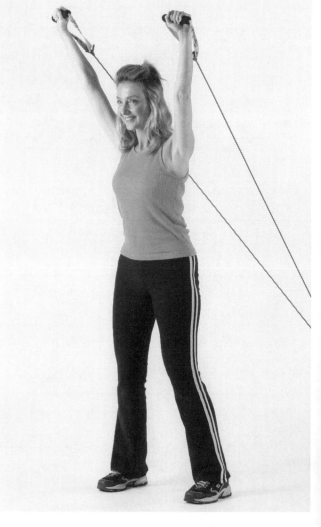

# Shoulder Lateral Raise

**This exercise can be performed with both the exercise band and tube.**

## TECHNIQUE & FORM

Anchor the band at the floor. Stand with your feet hip distance apart and your knees slightly bent. Hold the band with both hands, your palms facing inward. Lift your arms up to shoulder level.

### Paul's Pro Tip

Avoid lifting your arms higher than shoulder height as it can irritate the shoulder joint.

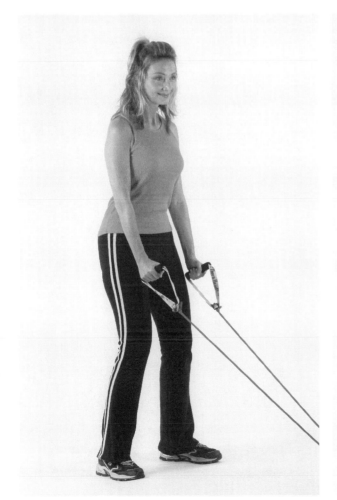

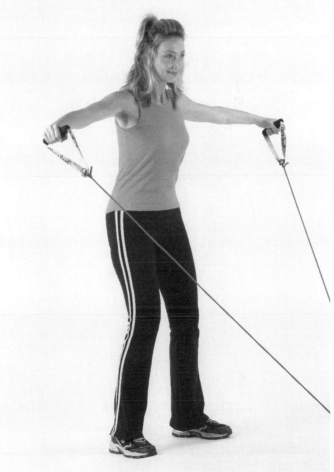

# Shoulder Front Raise

### TECHNIQUE & FORM
Anchor the band to the floor and hold it with both hands. Stand with your feet hip distance apart and your knees slightly bent. Your palms should face backwards. Lift your arms up to shoulder height.

*This exercise can be performed with both the exercise band and tube.*

*Paul's Pro Tip*
Keep your chest high and your shoulder back. Avoid rounding forward at your shoulders.

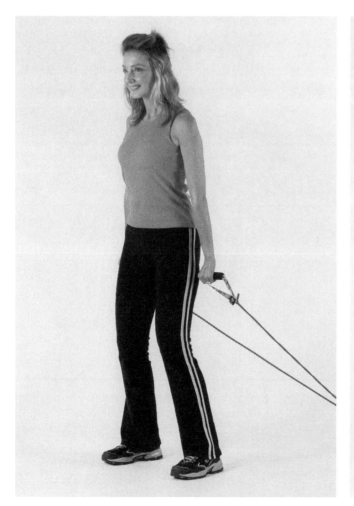
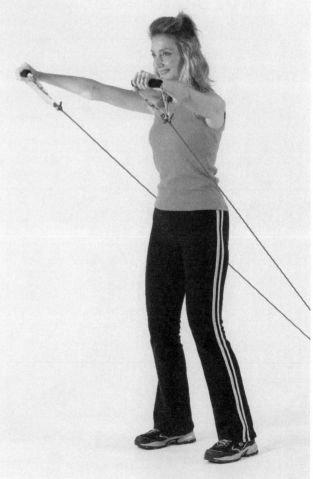

# Shoulder Rear Delt
## (Standing with Arms Extended)

### TECHNIQUE & FORM
Anchor the band at chest height. Stand with your feet in a staggered lunge position. Hold the band with both of your hands, your palms facing each other. Keeping your elbows slightly bent, extend your arms backward until they are parallel to your torso.

*This exercise can be performed with both the exercise band and tube.*

*Paul's Pro Tip*
This muscle is very hard to target, so it is best to begin this exercise with very light resistance, allowing precision in movement.

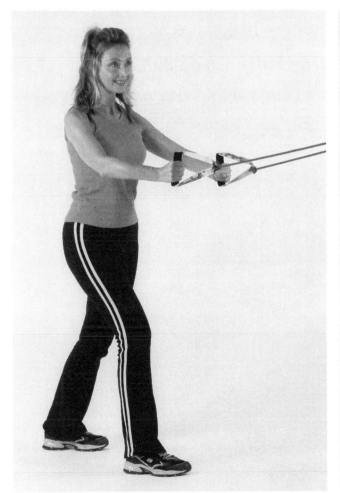
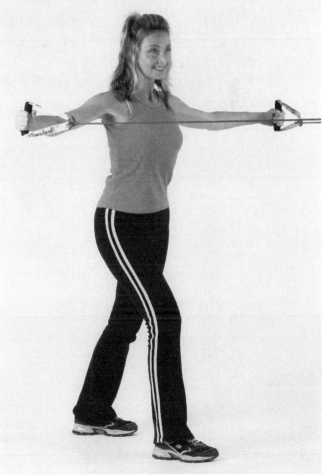

# *PowerBand* Back

***Trapezius, Latissimus Dorsi, Rhomboids, and Erectors***

You can't build a strong building without a strong foundation. Not only is your back the body's foundation, it's the basis of good posture.

## The Exercises

# Upper Back Standing Row

## (Elbows Lifted)

**This exercise can be performed with both the exercise band and tube.**

### TECHNIQUE & FORM
Anchor the band at chest height. Stand in a staggered lunge position. Hold the band with both of your hands, your palms facing the floor. Extend your arms to the front. Row back with your elbows held high.

### Paul's Pro Tip
Keep your torso upright and held still during the rowing movement.

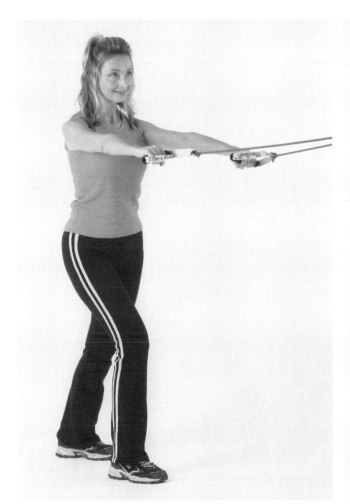
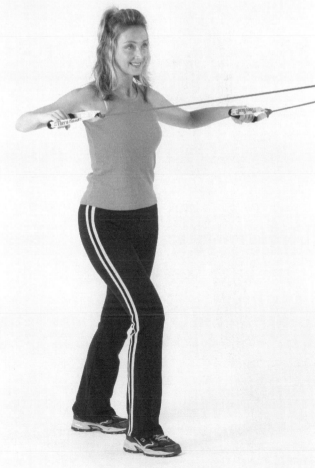

# Middle-Back Standing Row

*(Elbows by Waist)*

**This exercise can be performed with both the exercise band and tube.**

### TECHNIQUE & FORM
Anchor the band at chest height. Stand in a staggered lunge position. Hold the band with both of your hands, your palms facing the floor. Extend your arms to the front and row back with your elbows low and close to your waist.

**Paul's Pro Tip**

Focus on pinching your shoulder blades at the end point of the rowing movement.

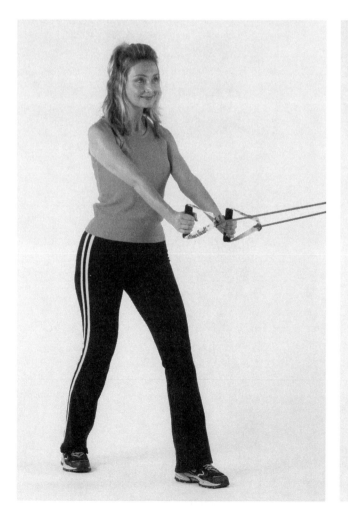
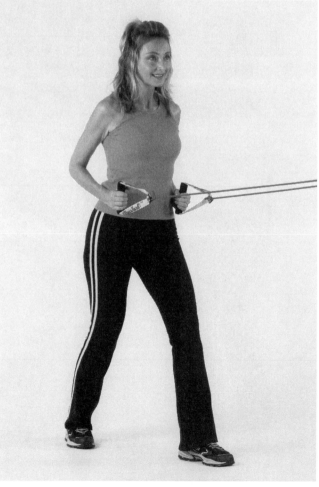

# Bent-Over Row

*This exercise can be performed with both the exercise band and tube.*

***Paul's Pro Tip***
Keep the natural arch in your lower back and your head in line with your spine. Draw your belly in toward your spine before executing this exercise.

## TECHNIQUE & FORM
Anchor the band at the floor. Stand with your feet shoulder width apart. Bend at your waist, holding the bands with both of your hands with palms facing each other. Row backward. Your elbows should slide past your ribs.

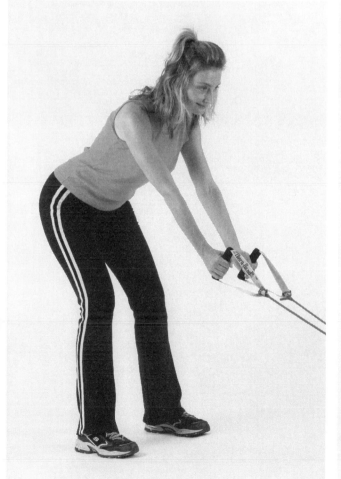

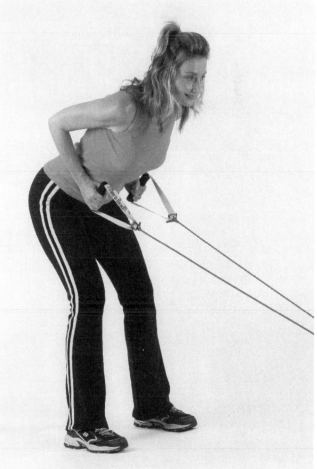

# Standing Lateral Straight Arm Pulldown

*This exercise can be performed with both the exercise band and tube.*

*Paul's Pro Tip*

Keep your elbow slightly bent. Pull your chest high while performing the downward press.

## TECHNIQUE & FORM

Anchor the band overhead. Stand with your feet shoulder width apart. Hold the band with both hands and extend your arms overhead with your palms facing the floor. Press your arms down past your hips.

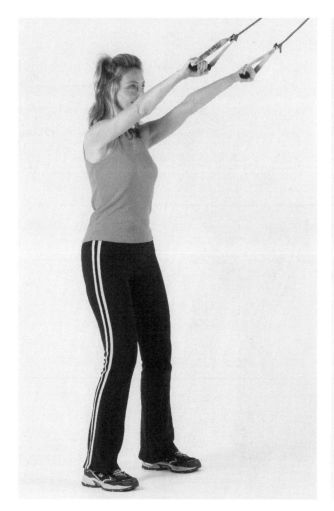
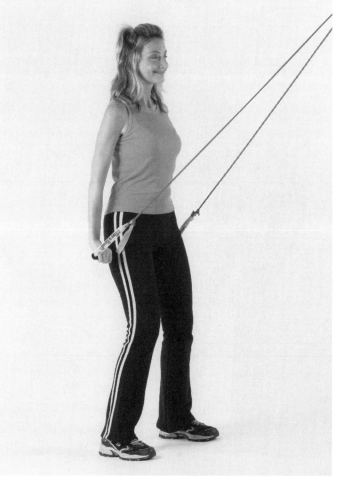

# Kneeling Lateral Pulldown

*This exercise can be performed with both the exercise band and tube.*

### Paul's Pro Tip

Changing the position of your hands so that your palms are facing towards you will intensify the exercise for your biceps.

## TECHNIQUE & FORM

Anchor the band overhead. Kneel on the floor. Hold the band in both hands, palms facing down. Pull down with your hands until your elbows touch the side of your ribs.

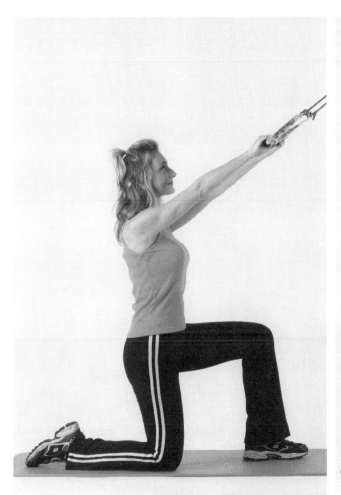
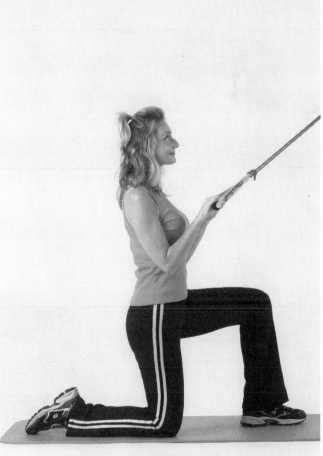

# Supine Lateral Pulldown on Ball

*This exercise can be performed with both the exercise band and tube.*

## TECHNIQUE & FORM

Anchor the band at the height of the ball. Begin in a bridge position with your head and shoulders resting comfortably on the ball. Have your knees, hips, and shoulders all in line with the floor, at the same height. Extend your arm overhead. Hold the band with both hands, palms facing the ceiling, and pull your elbows to your ribs.

### Paul's Pro Tip

You will need to engage your hamstrings, buttocks, and lower back while in this position.

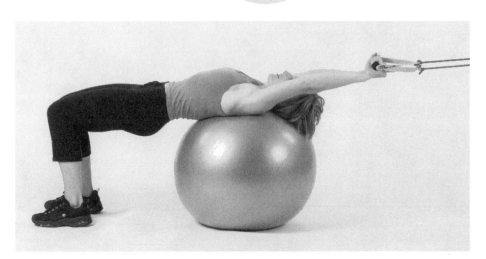

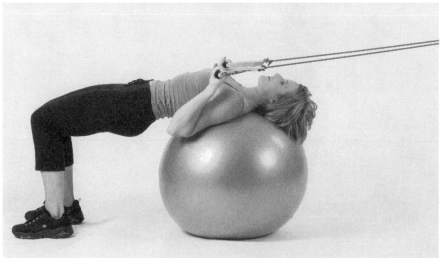

# Supine Lateral Pullover on Ball

*This exercise can be performed with both the exercise band and tube.*

### Paul's Pro Tip

Draw your shoulder blades down into their natural seated position before beginning this exercise.

## TECHNIQUE & FORM

Anchor the band at the height of the ball. Begin in a bridge position with your head and shoulders resting comfortably on the ball. Have your knees, hips, and shoulders all in line with the floor, at the same height. Extend your arms overhead. Hold the band with both hands, palms facing the ceiling. Keep your arms straight and pull the bands so that your palms come to the top of your thighs.

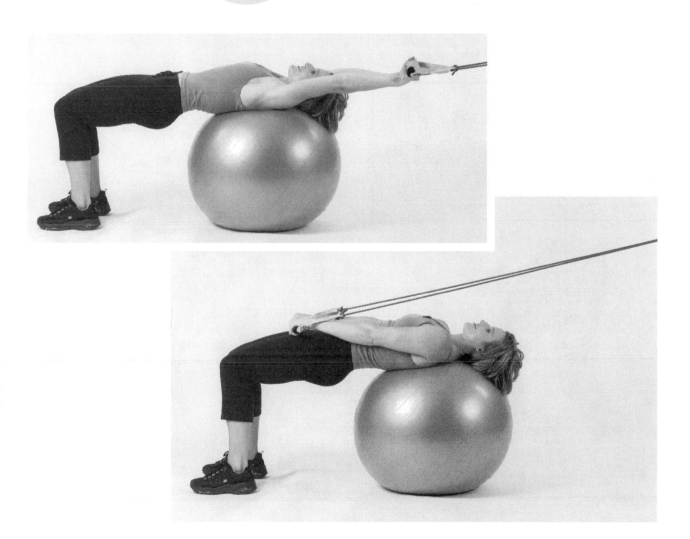

# Standing Lateral Pulldown

*This exercise can be performed with both the exercise band and tube.*

### Paul's Pro Tip

Avoid wasting energy by holding the bands tightly in your hands. Instead, allow the elbows to lead the way for the proper pathway of movement.

## TECHNIQUE & FORM

Anchor the band overhead. Stand with your feet in a staggered lunge position. Hold the band with both hands, extending your arms overhead with your palms facing away from your body. Pull down on the band until your elbows reach your ribs.

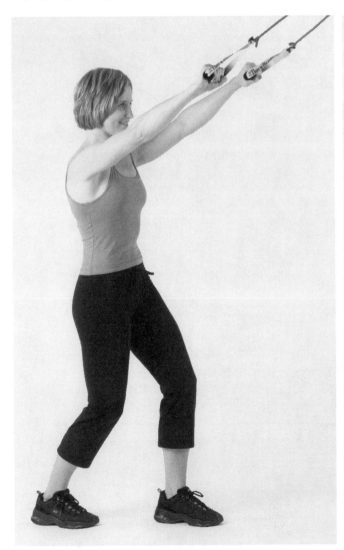
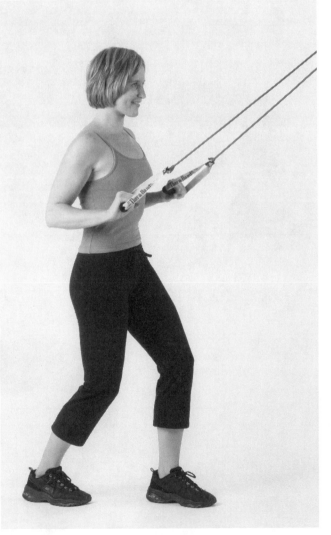

# Prone Lateral Pulldown on Ball

*This exercise can be performed with both the exercise band and tube.*

### Paul's Pro Tip
If you are using heavy resistance, the feet must be anchored by weights and/or an immobile object.

## TECHNIQUE & FORM
Anchor the band at ball height. Place your chest on the ball with your legs extended behind you. Extend your arms overhead and hold the band with both hands, your palms facing the floor. Pull down until your elbows reach your ribs.

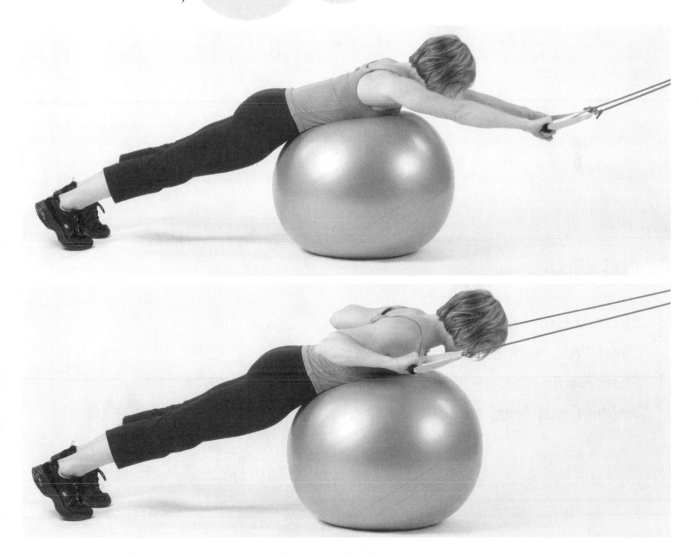

# *PowerBand* Chest

**Pectoralis Major and Pectoralis Minor**

Win the fight against gravity and keep your chest firm and taut. The chest muscles are responsible for any heavy pushing, and you can improve your posture greatly by exercising your pecs. Holding your chest high is one of the first steps toward good posture.

## The Exercises

**Chest Press with Tube,** *page 49*

**Chest Press with Band,** *page 50*

**Chest Fly Bungee,** *page 51*

**Incline Chest Press on Ball,** *page 52*

# Chest Press with Tube

*This exercise can only be performed with the exercise tube.*

### Paul's Pro Tip

Keeping your chest high and your shoulders back through the full range of movement will help target the chest muscles.

## TECHNIQUE & FORM

Anchor the bungee at chest height. Stand with your feet in a staggered position, your knees slightly bent. Hold bungee with both hands. Keep your elbows at a 90 degree angle from your torso. Press your hands forward until your arms are fully extended.

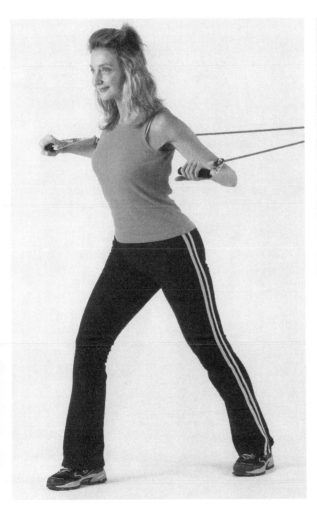
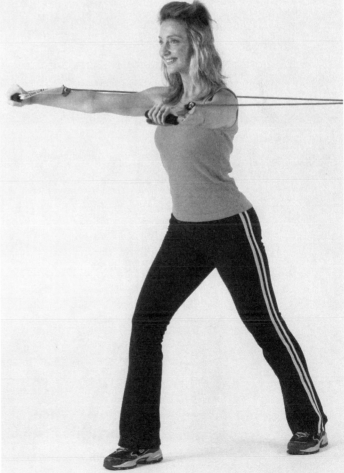

# Chest Press with Band

*This exercise can only be performed with the exercise band.*

## TECHNIQUE & FORM

Stand with your feet in a staggered position, your knees slightly bent. Wrap the band around your upper chest and under your arms. Hold with both hands and press forward with your hands.

### Paul's Pro Tip

Avoid rounding your shoulders forward and you will be better able to target the chest.

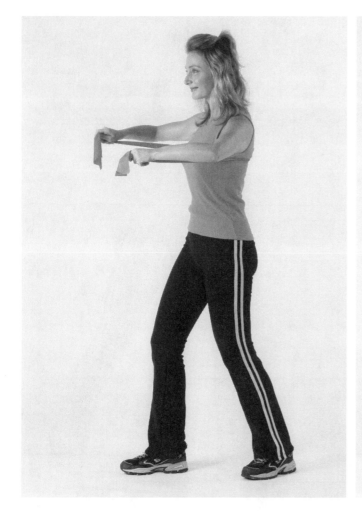
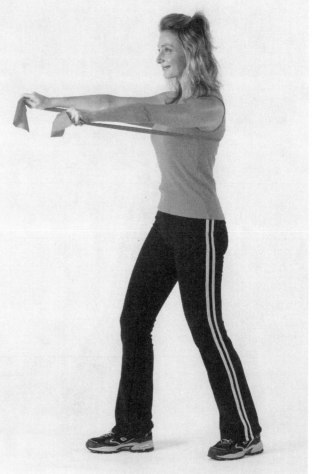

# Chest Fly Bungee

This exercise can be performed with both the exercise band and tube.

## TECHNIQUE & FORM

Anchor the bungee at chest height. Stand with your feet in a staggered position, your knees slightly bent. Hold band with both of your hands, arms extended to your sides. Keep your elbows slightly bent and draw your hands together.

### Paul's Pro Tip

Imagine wrapping your arms around a tree.

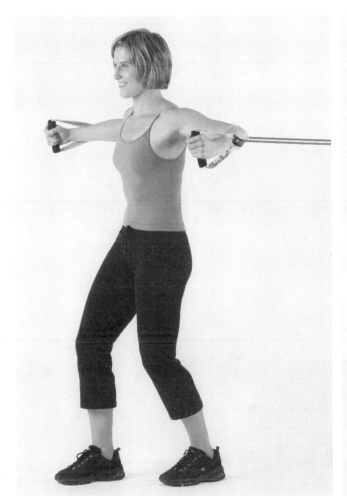
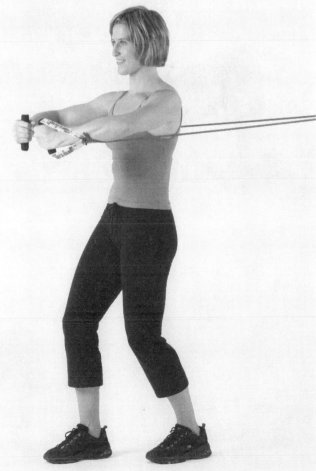

# Incline Chest Press on Ball

**TECHNIQUE & FORM**

Anchor the band at the floor. Sit on the floor with your knees bent and your mid-back against the ball. Hold band with both of your hands and press forward.

*This exercise can be performed with both the exercise band and tube.*

*Paul's Pro Tip*

To give the Incline Press more intensity, allow your elbows to reach back and touch the ball before pressing forward.

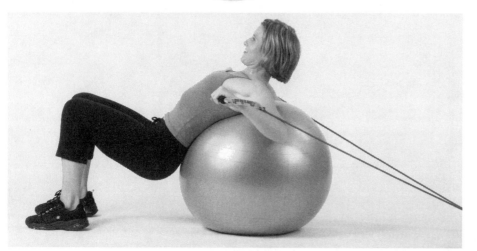

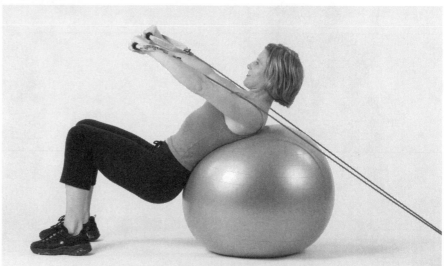

# PowerBand Abs

**Rectus Abdominis, External Obliques, and Internal Obliques**

Obsessed with lean, tight abs? So are most of us. Nothing speaks louder about your conditioning than strong abs. While the following exercises target your abs directly, you'll find that all of the exercises in the standing position will benefit your abs.

## The Exercises

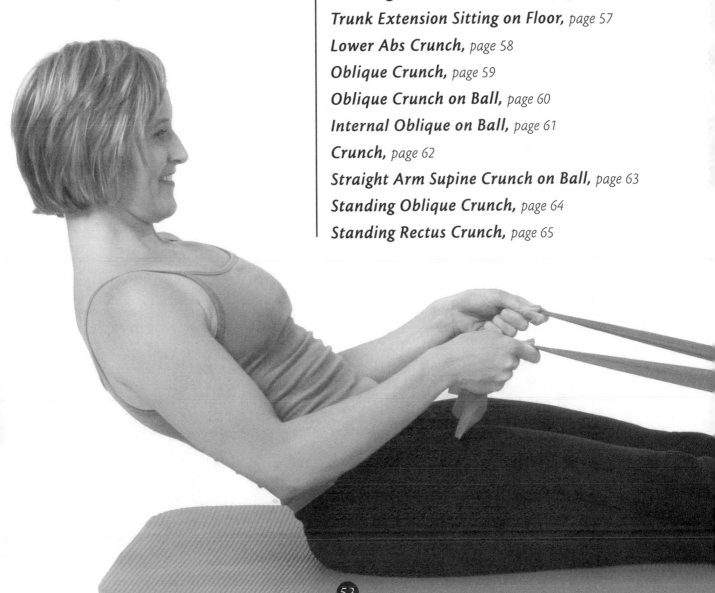

# Seated Rotation on Ball

## TECHNIQUE & FORM

Anchor the band overhead. Sit on apex of the ball with your feet flat on the floor. Hold the band in one hand, your palm on your shoulder. Now curl your shoulder toward your opposite hip.

*This exercise can be performed with both the exercise band and tube.*

### Paul's Pro Tip

Be careful not to slouch when seated on the ball. Initiate this by first bracing the abdominals.

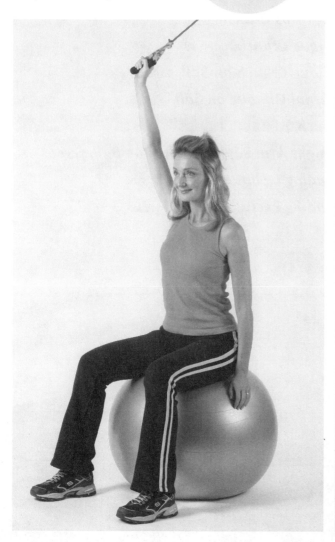 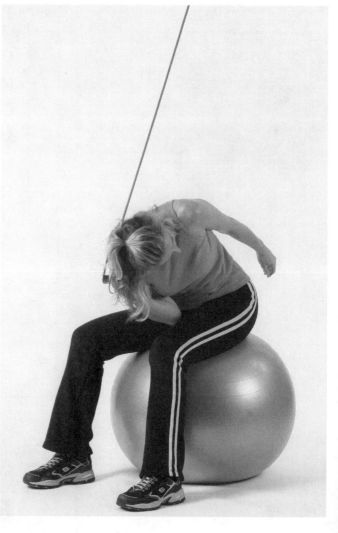

# Standing Side Bend

*(Hand by Waist)*

### TECHNIQUE & FORM

Anchor the band to the floor. Stand with your feet shoulder width apart, keeping your knees slightly bent. Hold band with one hand. Keep your arm straight, your chest high, and bend at your waist away from the anchor point.

*This exercise can be performed with both the exercise band and tube.*

*Paul's Pro Tip*

Keep your abdominals engaged and bend directly to the side, not rotating the trunk.

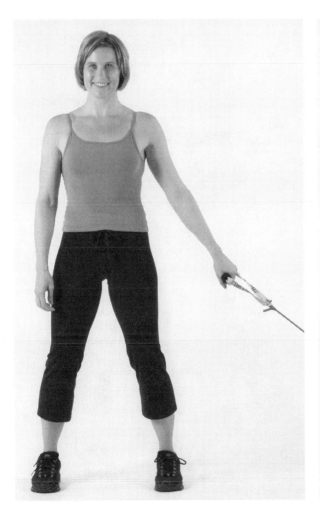
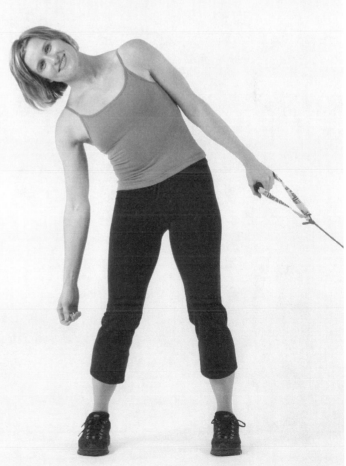

# Standing Overhead Side Bend
## (Hands Overhead)

### TECHNIQUE & FORM
Anchor the band overhead. Stand with your feet shoulder width apart, keeping your knees slightly bent. Hold the band with both hands, keeping your arms straight and your chest high. Bend laterally to the opposite side.

*This exercise can be performed with both the exercise band and tube.*

**Paul's Pro Tip**
The elbow should be in line with your ears.

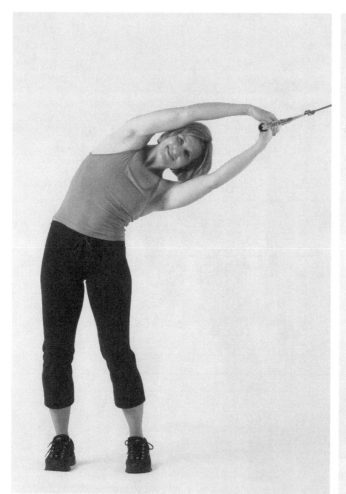
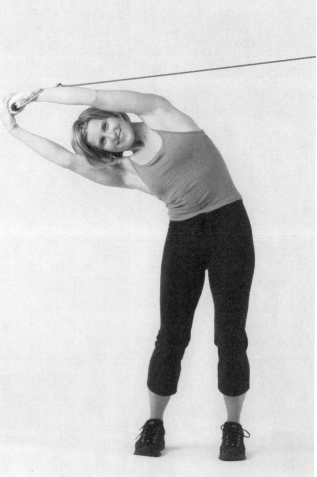

# Trunk Extension Sitting on Floor

*This exercise can be performed with both the exercise band and tube.*

### TECHNIQUE & FORM
Sit with your legs extended. Stretch the middle of the band around both of your feet and grasp both ends of the band with your hands at your chest. Lean back, stretching the band as you do. Keep your lumbar spine straight by extending at the hips. Slowly return to the starting position.

*Paul's Pro Tip*
Bend your knees if there is any strain in your lower back.

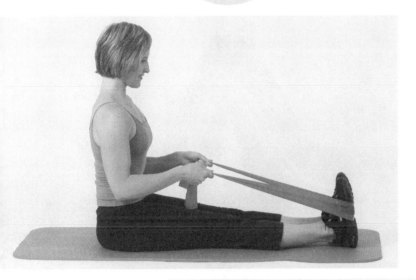

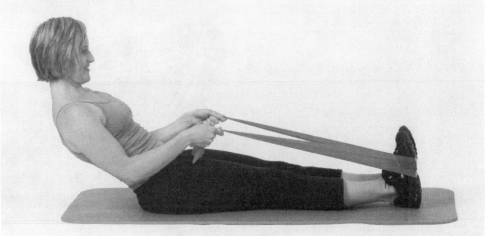

# Lower Abs Crunch

*This exercise can be performed with both the exercise band and tube.*

### TECHNIQUE & FORM
Lie on your back with your hips and knees flexed. Stretch the band over your knees and have it cross underneath. Secure each end of the band under your hands with elbows extended by your sides. Lift your knees upward, thus lifting your hips off the floor. Slowly return to the starting position.

*Paul's Pro Tip*
Keep your lower back firmly pressed to floor during the full range of exercise.

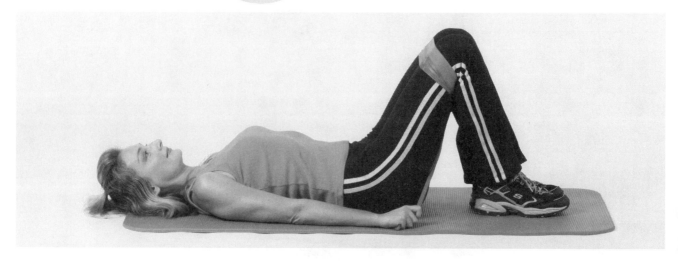

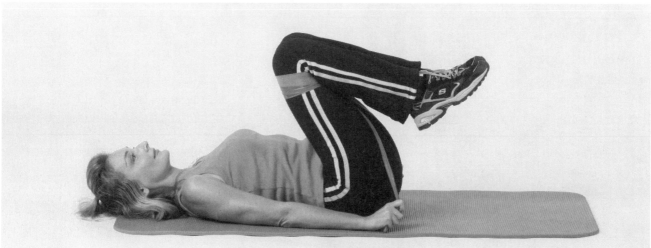

58

# Oblique Crunch

*This exercise can be performed with both the exercise band and tube.*

**TECHNIQUE & FORM**

Anchor the band at the floor. Lie on the floor with your knees bent. Hold it with one arm, extended over your chest. Draw your hand across your chest to the opposite hip.

*Paul's Pro Tip*

Extend your opposing arm to the side for more stability.

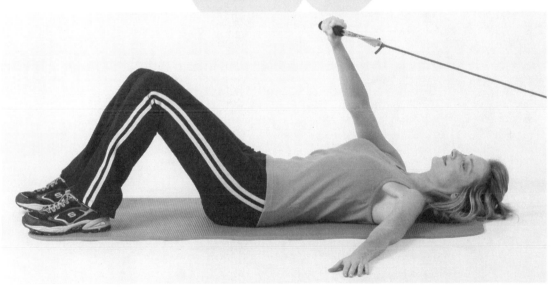

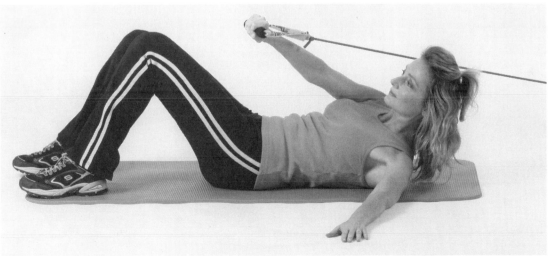

# Oblique Crunch on Ball

*This exercise can be performed with both the exercise band and tube.*

**Paul's Pro Tip**
Lower your hips on the ball if there is any stress in your lower back.

## TECHNIQUE & FORM

Anchor the band at the height of the ball. Lie on the ball in a bridge position with your lower back supported. Extend one arm over your chest and hold the band. Draw your hand toward the opposite hip.

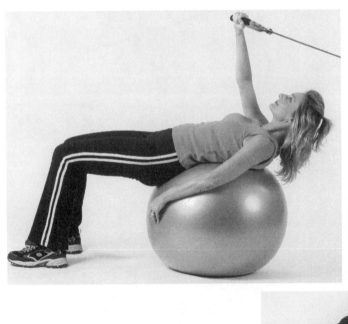

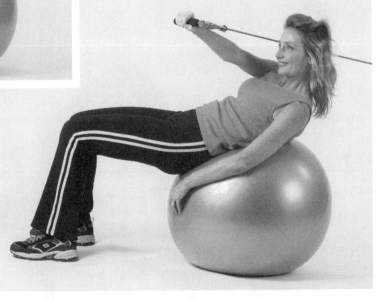

# Internal Oblique on Ball

*This exercise can be performed with both the exercise band and tube.*

**TECHNIQUE & FORM**

Anchor the band overhead. Place your waist on the ball with your feet spread wide for stability. Reach overhead with your arm and hold the band, bringing the top shoulder to hip on the same side.

*Paul's Pro Tip*

Place your lower hand on the floor or the ball for additional stability.

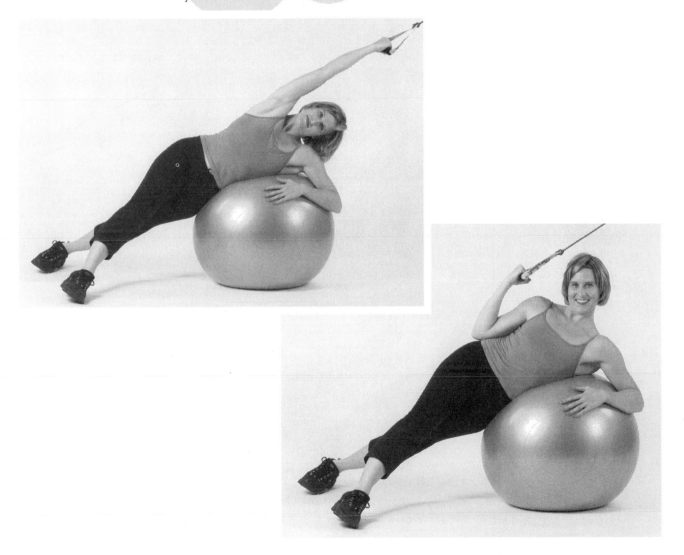

# Crunch

## TECHNIQUE & FORM

Securely attach the ends of the band to a stationary object near the floor. Lie on your back with your knees bent. Extend your arms in front and grasp the middle of the band with your hands close together. Keep your elbows straight in front and curl your trunk upward, lifting your shoulder blades from the floor.

*This exercise can be performed with both the exercise band and tube.*

*Paul's Pro Tip*

Tuck your chin to your chest to avoid neck strain.

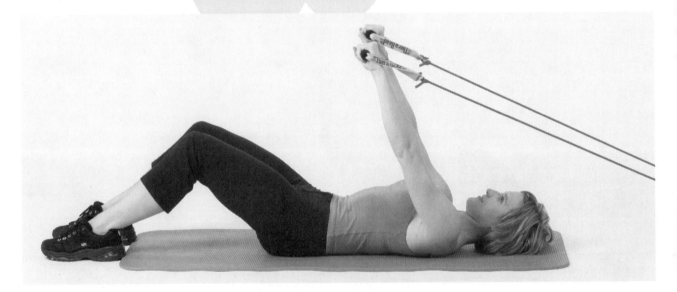

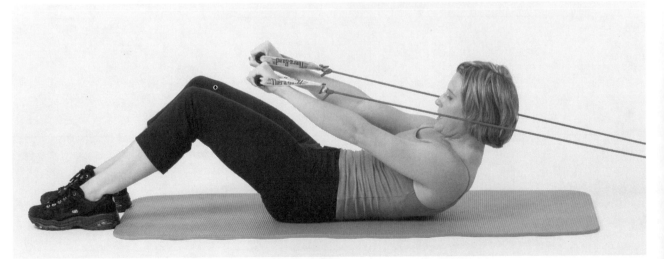

# Straight Arm Supine Crunch on Ball

*This exercise can be performed with both the exercise band and tube.*

### Paul's Pro Tip
Roll your shoulders off the ball, curling your rib cage to your hips.

## TECHNIQUE & FORM
The band should be anchored low on the floor. Lie with your lower back on the ball. Hold the band with both hands over your chest. Press forward, lifting your shoulder blades off the ball.

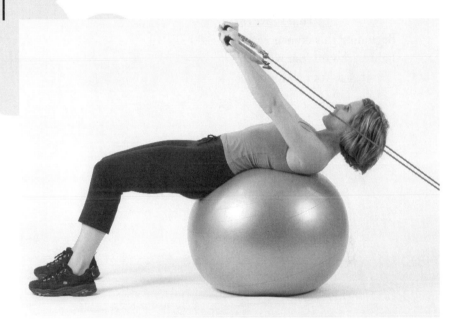

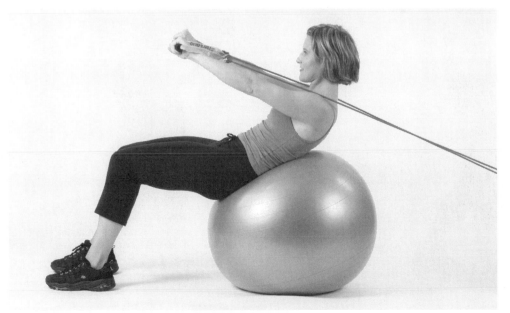

# Standing Oblique Crunch

*This exercise can be performed with both the exercise band and tube.*

### TECHNIQUE & FORM
Anchor band high. Stand in a staggered lunge position. Hold the band with one hand and place it, with your palm facing down, on your shoulder. Now, rotate your shoulder down toward your opposite hip.

### Paul's Pro Tip
Beginning this crunch with a slight backward lean will help engage your abdominals.

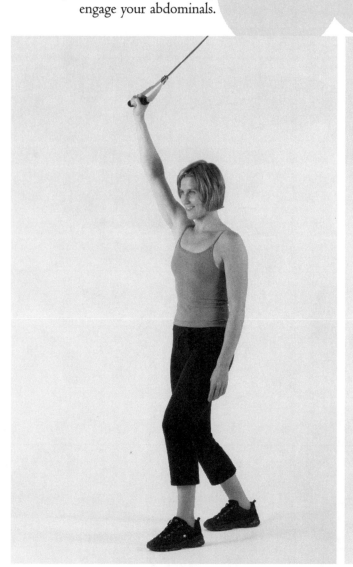
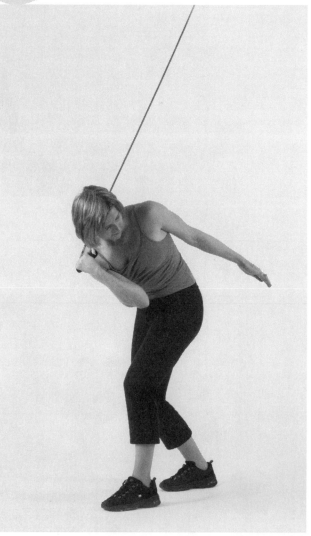

# Standing Rectus Crunch

*This exercise can be performed with both the exercise band and tube.*

**Paul's Pro Tip**
Tuck your chin to your chest before crunching down.

## TECHNIQUE & FORM
Anchor band high. Stand in staggered lunge position. Hold the band with both hands and place your hands, palms facing down, on your shoulders. Crunch down toward your hips.

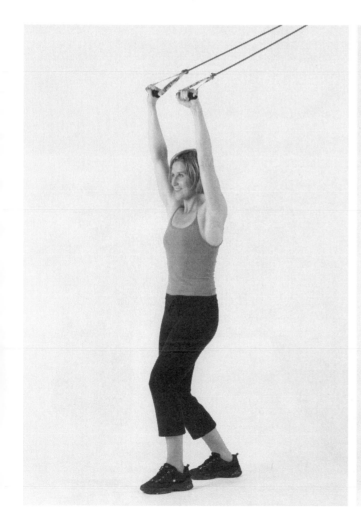
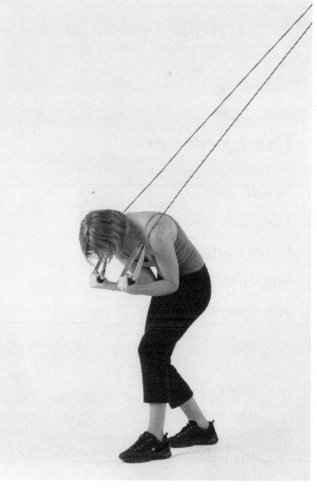

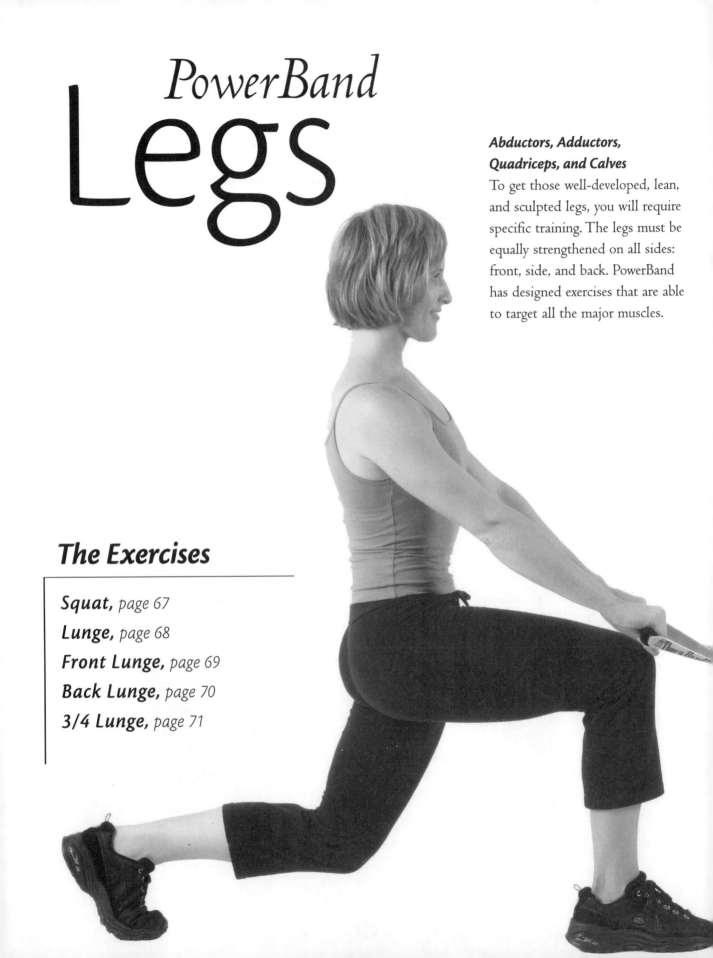

# *PowerBand*
# Legs

**Abductors, Adductors, Quadriceps, and Calves**

To get those well-developed, lean, and sculpted legs, you will require specific training. The legs must be equally strengthened on all sides: front, side, and back. PowerBand has designed exercises that are able to target all the major muscles.

## The Exercises

# Squat

*This exercise can only be performed with the exercise band.*

### Paul's Pro Tip

If you're having problems with form, practice by standing in front of a chair and dropping your butt backward until it touches the seat. Then return to the starting position. Maintain the arch in your lower back throughout the full exercise.

## TECHNIQUE & FORM

Stand on the band with both feet. Stand with your feet shoulder width apart and your knees bent at a 90 degree angle. Hold the band with both hands, your arms to the side. Rise up to standing position.

## VARIATION

The Squat can also be performed with the tube. To do so, anchor the band to the floor and stand with your feet shoulder width apart and your knees bent at a 90 degree angle. Hold the band in both hands and extend your arms in front of torso. Rise to a standing position.

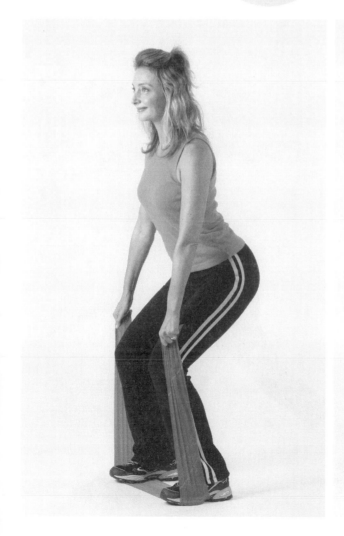
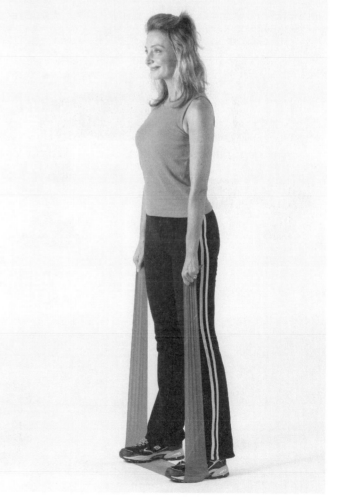

# Lunge

*This exercise can be performed with both the exercise band and tube.*

*Paul's Pro Tip*
Avoid banging the rear knee on the floor while in the lowered position.

## TECHNIQUE & FORM
Anchor the bungee at the floor and hold it with both hands, arms extended toward the floor. Stand in a staggered deep lunge position. Your front thigh should be parallel to the floor with your knee bent at 90 degrees, and your back leg should be bent with your knee a few inches from the floor. Rise up to a standing position.

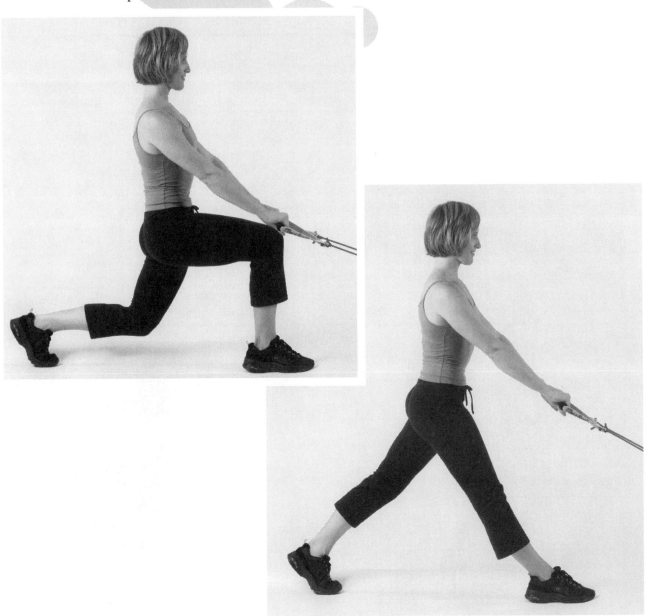

# Front Lunge

### TECHNIQUE & FORM
Stand in a staggered deep lunge position, with your front thigh parallel to the floor with your knee bent at 90 degrees, and your back leg bent with your knee a few inches from the floor. Your front foot should stand on the band. Hold the band in both hands with your arms at your side. Rise up to a standing position.

*This exercise can only be performed with the exercise band.*

*Paul's Pro Tip*
Keep your front knee directly over your ankle and do not allow it to creep over the toes.

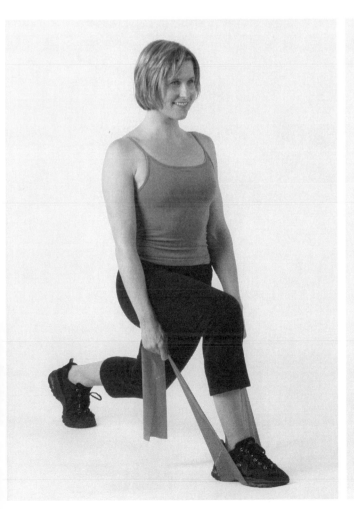
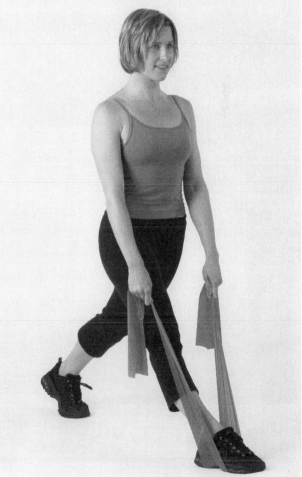

# Back Lunge

## TECHNIQUE & FORM

Anchor the band at chest height. Hold it with both hands, arms extended to the front. Stand with your feet hip distance apart. Step back with one leg into a lunge, then return to the starting position.

*This exercise can be performed with both the exercise band and tube.*

*Paul's Pro Tip*

Return to the starting position in a controlled movement. You should resist the temptation of allowing the band to assist you.

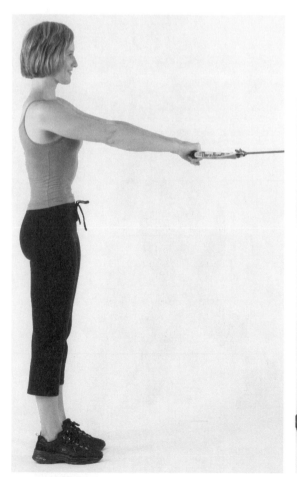

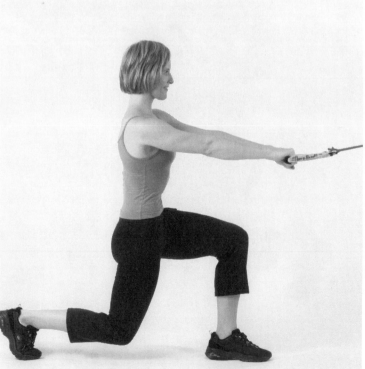

# 3/4 Lunge

*This exercise can be performed with both the exercise band and tube.*

### TECHNIQUE & FORM
Anchor the band at chest height. Stand with your feet hip distance apart. Hold the band with both of your hands with your arms extended out. Step back with one leg into a 3/4 lunge position.

*Paul's Pro Tip*

Try experimenting with different angles and directions of the lunge to target different muscle fibers of the leg. This also will help you improve your balance.

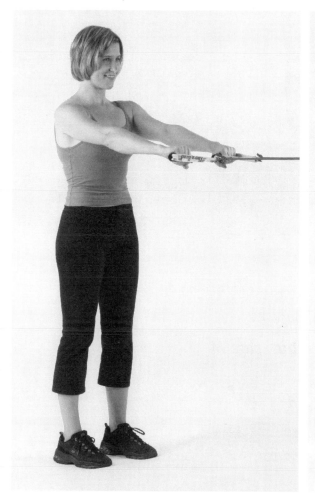 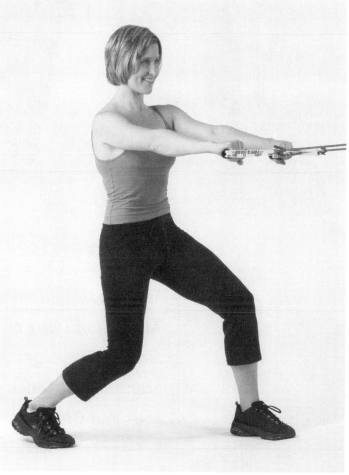

# *PowerBand*
# Glutes

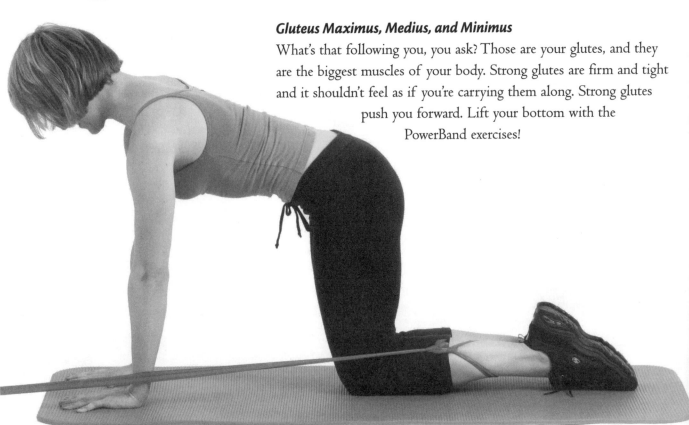

### Gluteus Maximus, Medius, and Minimus

What's that following you, you ask? Those are your glutes, and they are the biggest muscles of your body. Strong glutes are firm and tight and it shouldn't feel as if you're carrying them along. Strong glutes push you forward. Lift your bottom with the PowerBand exercises!

## The Exercises

# Standing Abduction

## TECHNIQUE & FORM

Anchor the band at the floor. Stand with your feet hip distance apart. Tie the other end of the band around the ankle of your outside leg. Keep your hips squared as you lift your leg to the side.

*This exercise can only be performed with the exercise band.*

*Paul's Pro Tip*
Use a chair for stability if you are unable to maintain good balance.

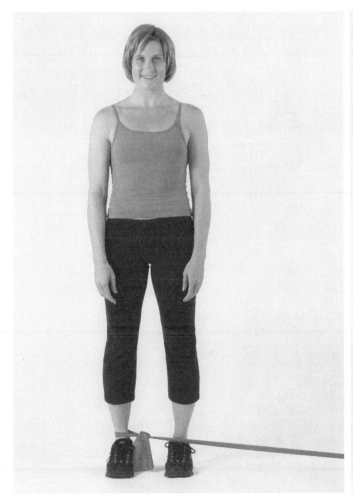
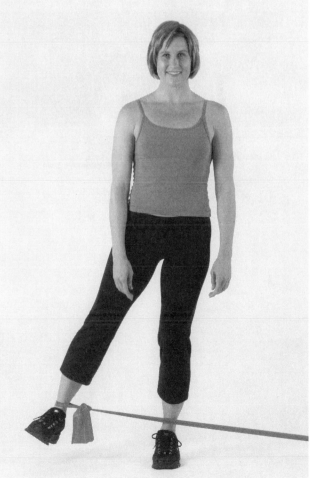

# Abduction Lying on Floor

*This exercise can only be performed with the exercise band.*

*Paul's Pro Tip*
Finding a comfortable seated position and remembering to engage your abs will help avoid stress on your lower back.

## TECHNIQUE & FORM
Anchor the band at the floor. Sit on the floor. Tie the other end of the band around the leg of your inside ankle. Bending the knee of other leg, draw the leg with the band to the midline of your body.

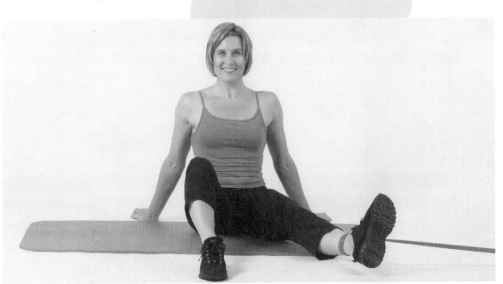

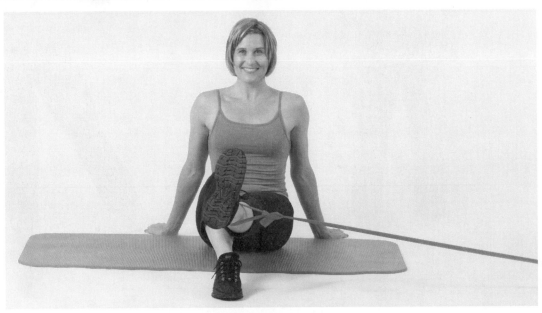

# Side Shuffle
## (Band on Ankle)

### TECHNIQUE & FORM
Anchor band at the floor. Stand with your feet hip distance apart. Tie the other end of the band around the ankle of your inside leg. Keep your hips squared and draw your leg towards the midline of your body.

*This exercise can only be performed with the exercise band.*

*Paul's Pro Tip*
Keep constant tension on the band to make this exercise more effective.

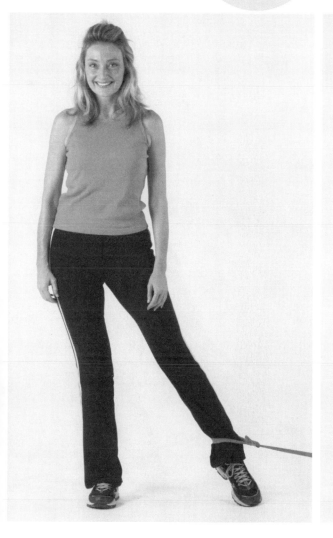
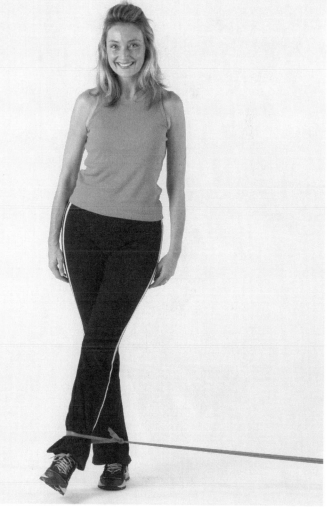

# Standing Glutes

## TECHNIQUE & FORM
Stand with your feet hip distance apart and the band anchored to the floor. Tie the other end of the band around your ankle. Bend your knees and extend your leg backwards.

*This exercise can only be performed with the exercise band.*

*Paul's Pro Tip*
Keep your hips squared and do not rotate from side to side. Use a wall or a chair to help maintain your balance if necessary.

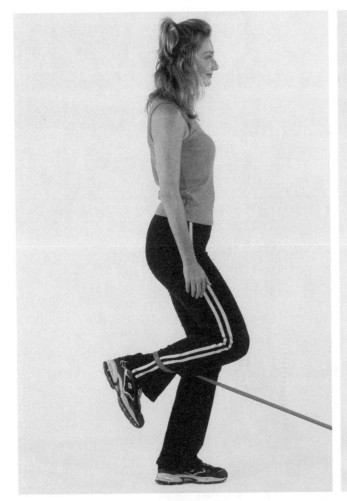
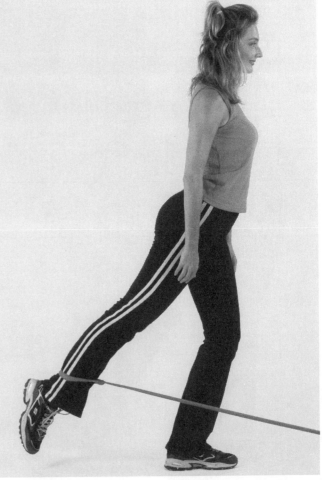

# Four Ped Glutes

This exercise can only be performed with the exercise band.

## TECHNIQUE & FORM
Anchor the band to the floor and tie the band around one of your ankles. Position your body on the floor with your hands under your shoulders and your knees under your hips. Extend the leg out so that it is in line with your torso. Return to the starting position with your knees next to each other.

**Paul's Pro Tip**
Place a towel under the knee remaining on the floor.

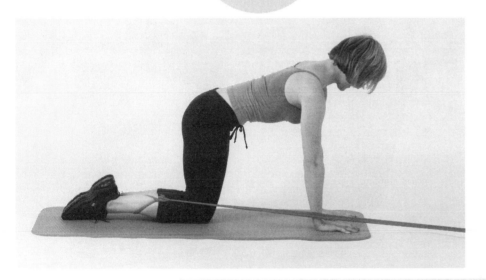

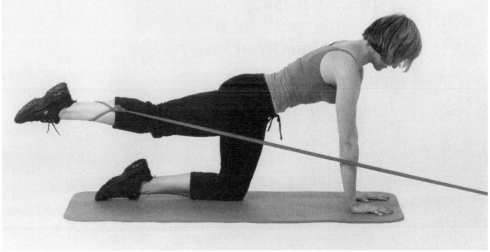

# *PowerBand* Hamstrings

**Biceps Femoris, Semitendinosus, Semimembranosus**

The hamstrings assist your glutes and are perhaps the most important muscle group in maintaining healthy knees. They have a tendency of becoming tight when they are weak, so try the following exercises designed with your flexibility in mind.

## The Exercises

# Standing Hamstring

**This exercise can only be performed with the exercise band.**

## TECHNIQUE & FORM

Anchor the band at the floor. Stand with your feet hip distance apart. Tie the other end of the band around your ankle. Extend your leg behind your hips without bending your knee.

***Paul's Pro Tip***

Avoid swinging your leg back by controlling the backward movement.

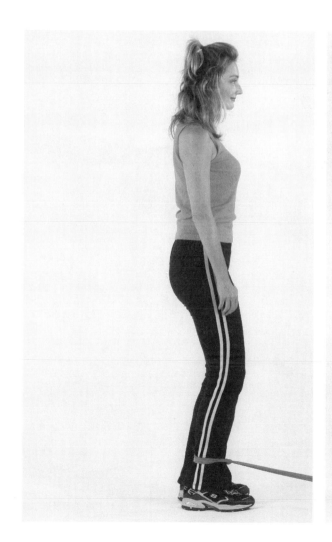
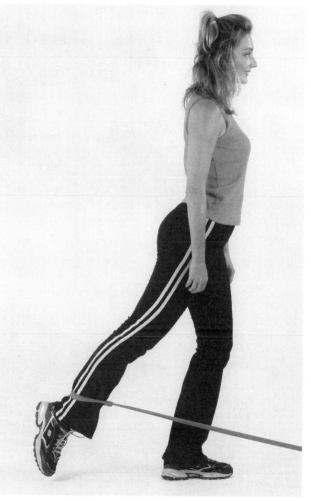

# Four Ped Hamstring

*This exercise can only be performed with the exercise band.*

## TECHNIQUE & FORM
Anchor the band to the floor and tie the band around one of your ankles. Position your body on the floor with your hands under your shoulders and your knees under your hips. Extend your leg out so that it is parallel to your torso. Keep your leg straight and lower it to the floor.

*Paul's Pro Tip*
Keep your abs tight and the leg straight at the knees.

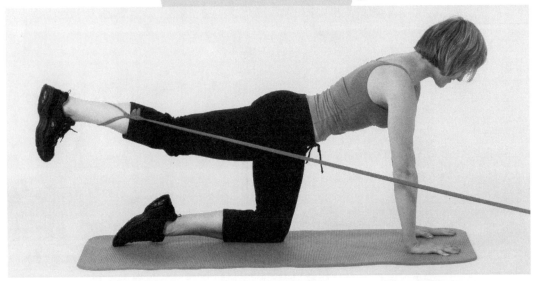

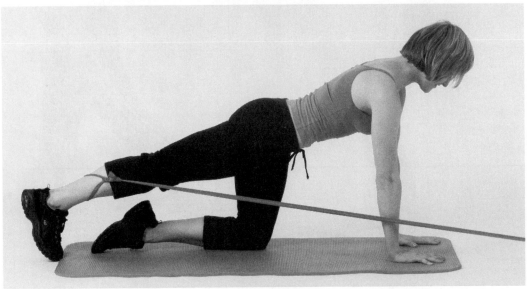

# Supine Hamstring

**TECHNIQUE & FORM**
Lie on the floor. Wrap one end of the band around your ankle. Hold the other end of the band with both of your hands. Lift leg to a 90 degree angle with the floor, then draw your leg down to the floor.

*This exercise can only be performed with the exercise band.*

*Paul's Pro Tip*
Keep your knee straight and your hips squared.

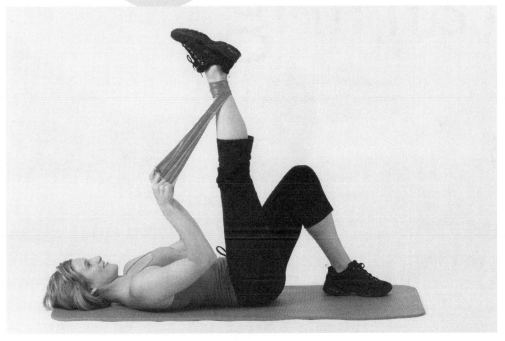

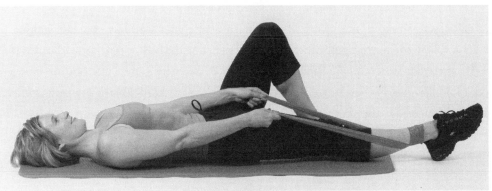

### Chapter 5

# PowerBand Flexibility Training

If you want to get the most out of your workout, flexibility training is a must. The benefits are endless, and if you plan on living actively and pain-free, the next few pages could change your life. Flexibility training will improve your balance, poor postural habits, and sports performance. Flexibility will make your body happy. So what are you waiting for?

If you're like most people, you might be confused on when and how to stretch properly. First off, you need to stretch after your workout, not before. If you strech before your workout, you risk injuring yourself. Before you workout, follow the warm-up provided, as it is designed with the PowerBand workout in mind..

Directly after your workout, you need to spend at least 5 minutes stretching out the muscles that you have just used. Hold the stretches for 10 to 20 seconds and be sure to keep breathing deeply and evenly. Stretching may feel a little uncomfortable, but never painful. If at any time you feel pain, stop what you are doing.

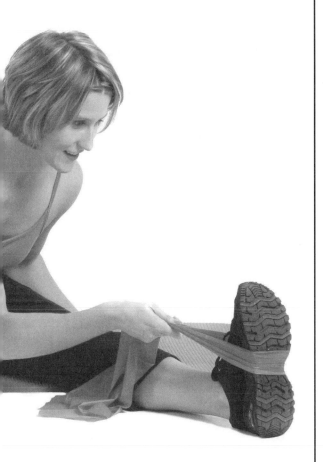

## The Exercises

# Chest Stretch

## TECHNIQUE & FORM
Kneel on the floor with the ball parallel to your shoulder. Bend your arm at a 90 degree angle and position the ball between your elbow and shoulder, pressing your chest gently toward the floor.

### *Paul's Pro Tip*
Moving the ball to different angles will stretch different areas of your chest.

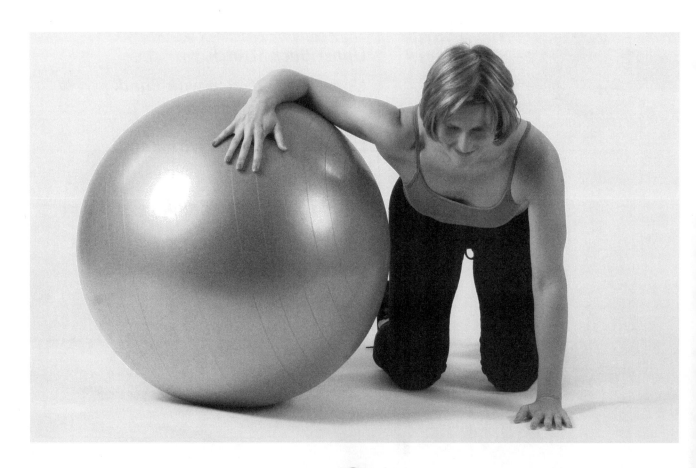

# Chest Stretch with Band

### TECHNIQUE & FORM

Hold the band in front of your chest with your arms held wide. Lift your arms over your head and hold them behind your shoulders.

***Paul's Pro Tip***

Begin conservatively, with hands held very wide. The narrower your grip on the band, the deeper the stretch will be.

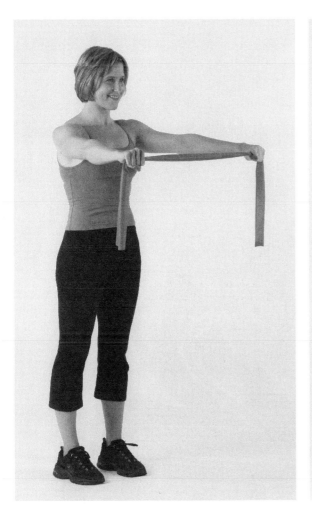
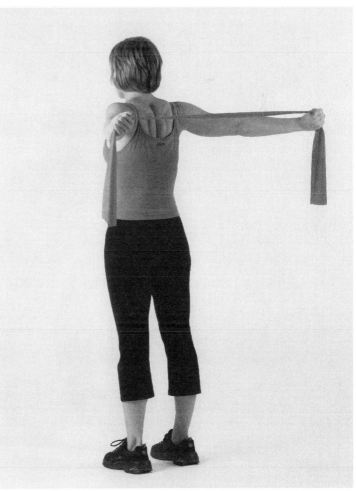

# Triceps Stretch

## TECHNIQUE & FORM

Kneel in front of the ball and place the back of one of your arms on the ball with the palm of your hand facing your shoulder. Press your chest toward the floor.

***Paul's Pro Tip***

Increasing the range of motion in this stretch will also target the lats.

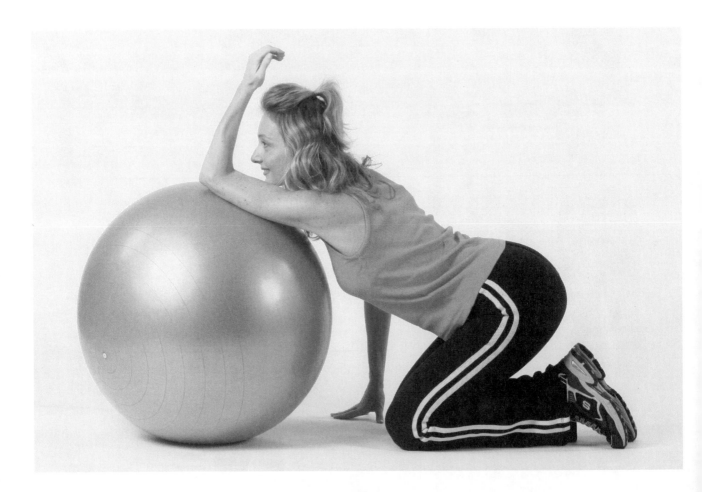

# Triceps Stretch with Band

## TECHNIQUE & FORM
Hold the band with both hands. Lift one hand overhead and move the other behind your back. Pull the band with your lower hand and bend your top arm at the elbow

**Paul's Pro Tip**
Keep elbow of the upper arm pointed upward.

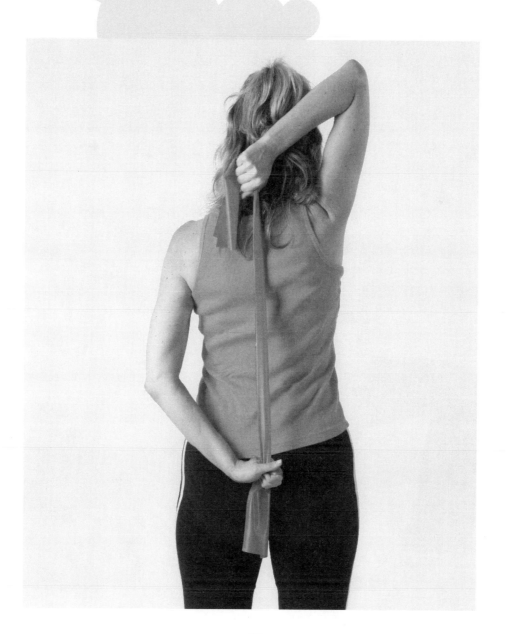

# Quadriceps Stretch

## TECHNIQUE & FORM

Place one knee on the floor with the instep on the ball. Be sure that the other knee is bent at 90 degrees with the knee directly over the ankle. Begin with your hands on the floor. As you become more flexible, place your hands on the bent knee or on your waist.

*Paul's Pro Tip*

To increase the stretch, press the hips away from the ball.

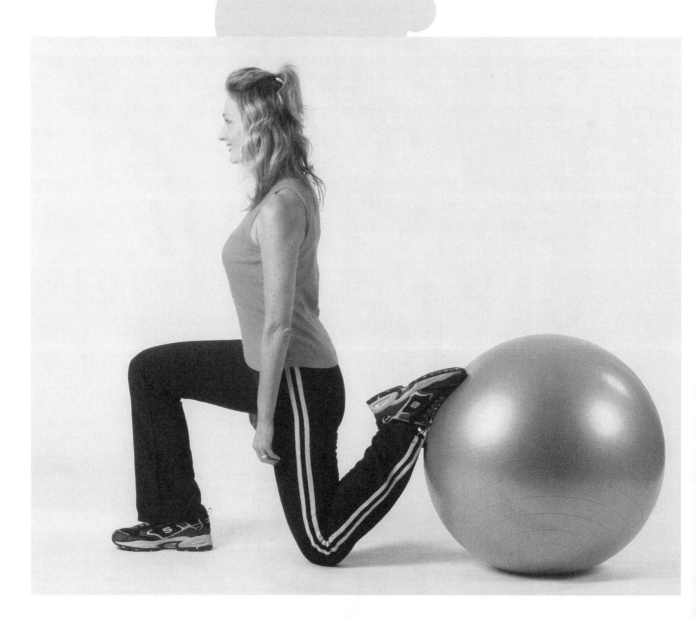

# Quadriceps Stretch with Band

***Paul's Pro Tip***

Increase the stretch of your quadriceps by actively flexing the hamstring muscles.

### TECHNIQUE & FORM

Place one knee on the floor and bend your other knee at 90 degrees. Wrapping the rear foot with the band, hold the band over your shouldler with the hand on the same side as the foot. Pull the band, lifting the rear foot off of the floor.

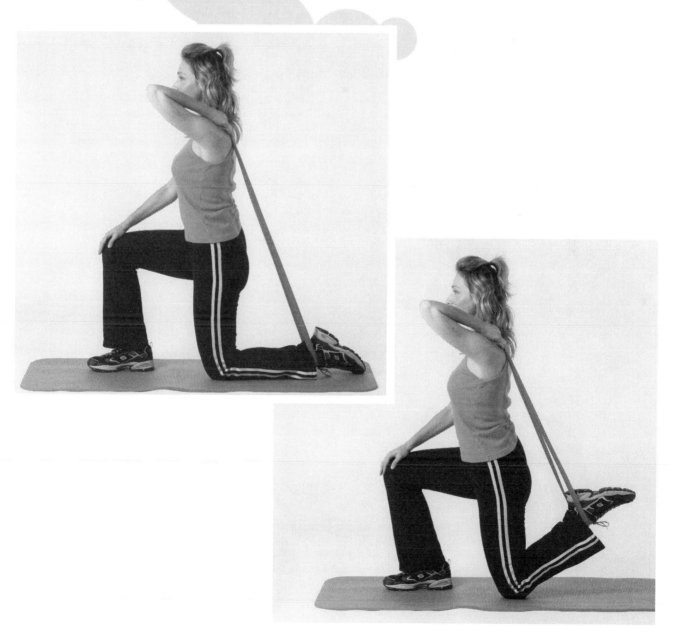

# Hamstring Stretch

### TECHNIQUE & FORM

Sit on the apex of the ball with your knees bent at 90-degree angle and your feet flat on floor. Push back on your heels, straightening your legs by bending forward at your hips and reaching hands toward feet.

### Paul's Pro Tip

Keeping the arch in the your lower back will help to target the back of your legs. Increase the stretch by flexing your toes back towards your hands.

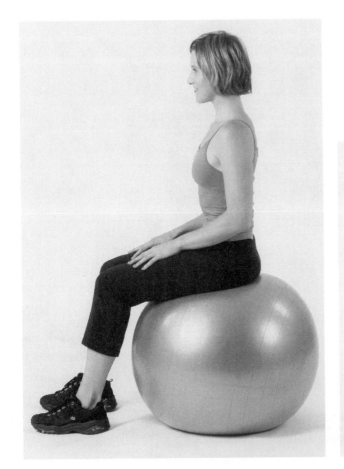

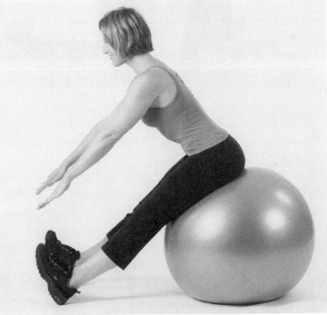

# Hamstring Stretch with Band

### TECHNIQUE & FORM
Lay on the floor with the band wrapped around one of your ankles. Hold the other end of the bands with your hands. Lift your leg and assist the stretch by pulling the leg toward your chest.

*Paul's Pro Tip*

Keep your leg as straight as possible and increase the stretch of the hamstring by flexing the front of your leg when performing the stretch.

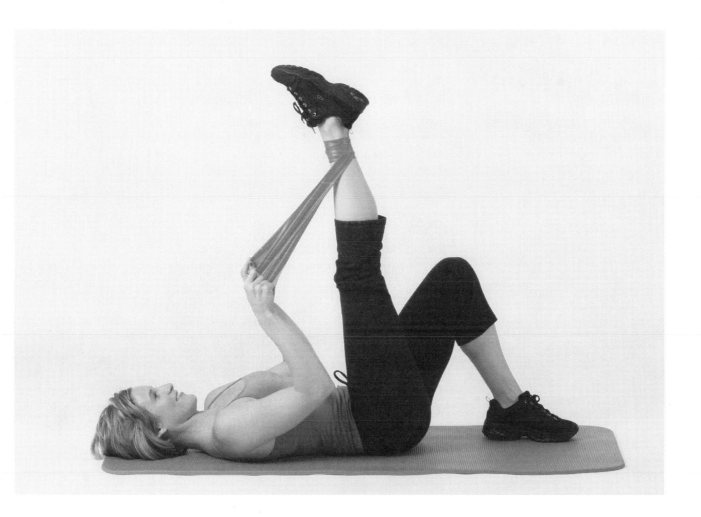

# Shoulder Stretch

**Paul's Pro Tip**
Roll the ball gently from left to right to stretch different muscles fibers. This also stretches the lats.

## TECHNIQUE & FORM

Kneel in front of the ball and place both of your hands on top of the ball with your arms extended. Press your chest toward the floor.

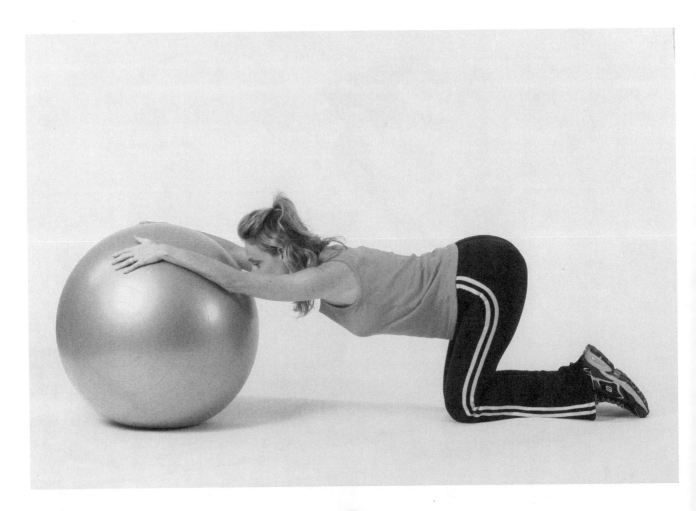

# Shoulder Stretch with Band

### Paul's Pro Tip
Keeping your palms facing your thighs will best target the shoulders. If you face your palms forward while doing this stretch, you will also stretch your biceps.

### TECHNIQUE & FORM
Anchor the band at floor level. Hold the band with your hands down by your hips. Step forward until you feel the stretch in the front of your shoulders.

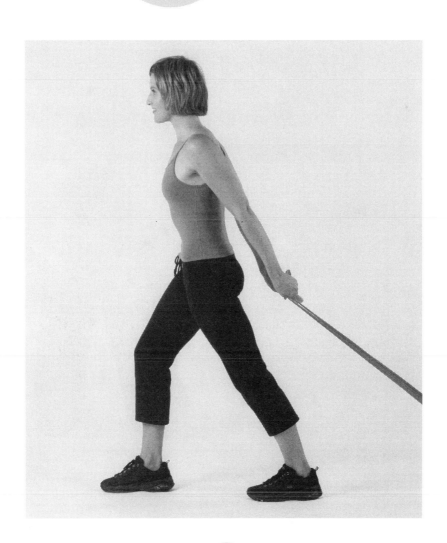

# Biceps Stretch

### TECHNIQUE & FORM
Kneel on the floor, extend your arm, and place your hand on the ball. Gently press your chest towards the floor.

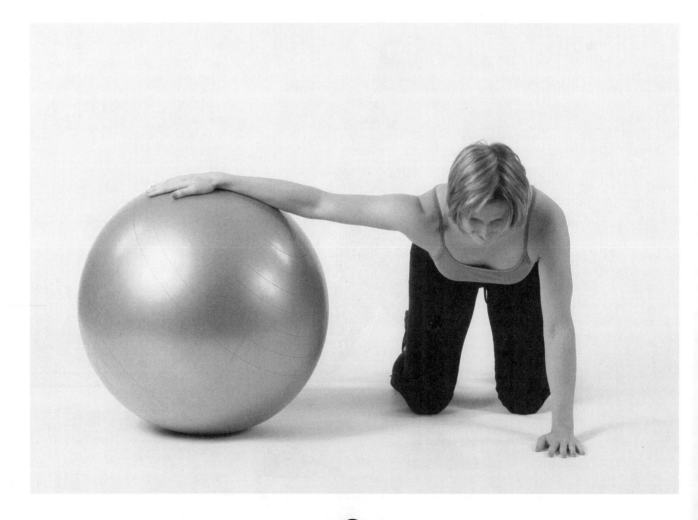

# Biceps Stretch with Band

*Paul's Pro Tip*

Keeping your shoulders down and relaxed will allow a better stretch in the biceps.

## TECHNIQUE & FORM

Anchor the band at shoulder height. Hold the band with both hands and extend your arms out to the side. Step forward until you feel a stretch in your biceps.

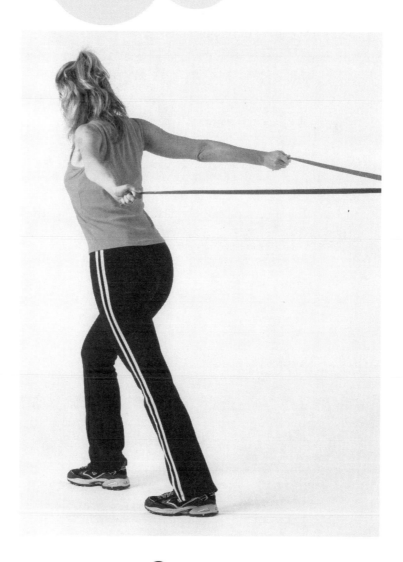

# Upper Back Stretch

### TECHNIQUE & FORM
Kneel in front of the ball with one arm between your chest and the ball. Press your chest forward.

*Paul's Pro Tip*

Move your arm around to target different muscle fibers.

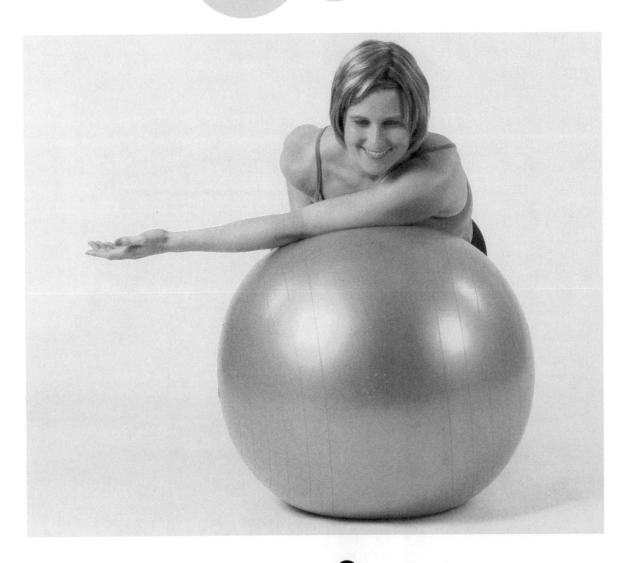

# Upper Back Stretch with Band

*Paul's Pro Tip*

Anchoring the band at different levels will target different parts of your shoulder.

## TECHNIQUE & FORM

Anchor the band at shoulder height. Cross one arm across your chest and hold the band with the outstretched hand. Turn your torso away from the band.

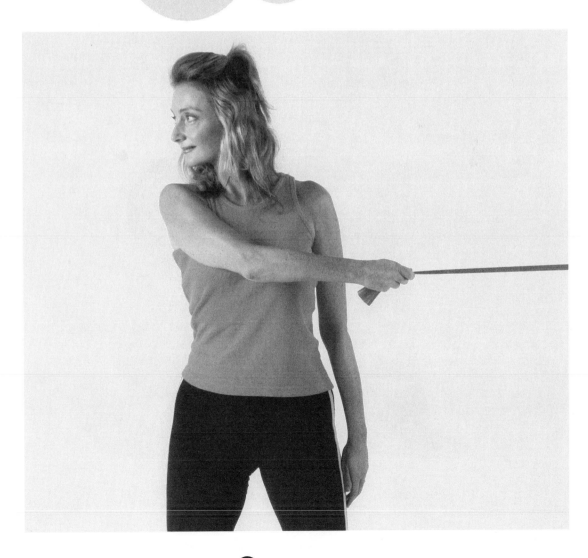

# Lower Back Stretch

***Paul's Pro Tip***

Make sure to keep the neck and
shoulders relaxed while you
increase the stretch by exhaling
slowly. Roll back up to the
starting position slowly with
your head finishing last.

## TECHNIQUE & FORM

Sit on the apex of the ball with your feet shoulder width apart
and flat on the floor. Draw your belly in tight and lower your head
between your knees, reaching your hands toward the floor.

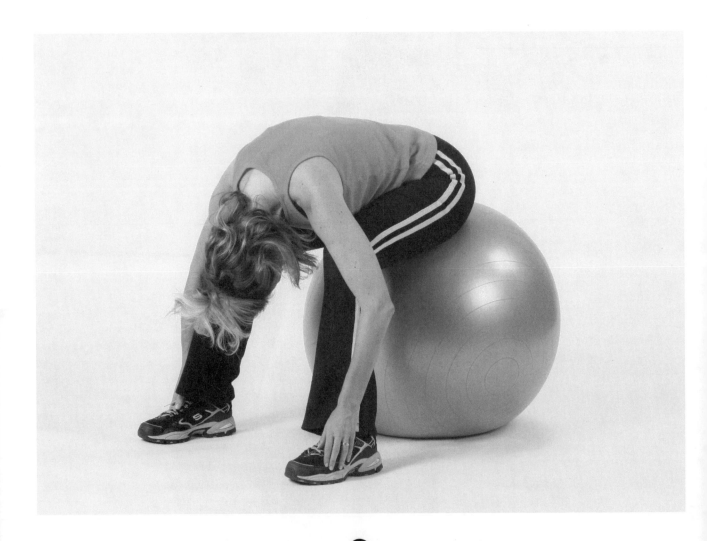

# Lower Back Stretch with Band

### TECHNIQUE & FORM
Sit on the floor with your legs extended. Place the band around your feet and hold the ends with both hands. As you exhale, reach your hands toward your feet, allowing the band to assist in the stretch.

*Paul's Pro Tip*

If you have tight hamstrings, try keeping your knees bent in this stretch.

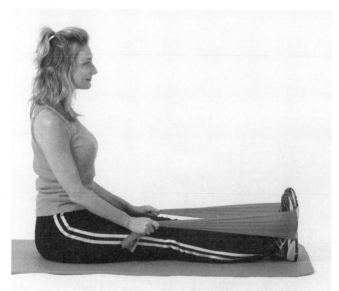

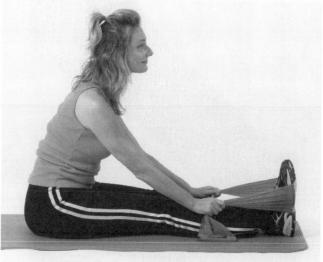

# Waist Stretch

## TECHNIQUE & FORM

Sit on the apex of the ball and roll down toward your lower back. Rotate on your side. Reach your top hand over your head and place your lower hand on the floor, keeping your feet wide for stability.

### Paul's Pro Tip

Placing your top leg behind the ball will help target the front of your waist. Placing your top leg in front of the ball will help target the back of your waist.

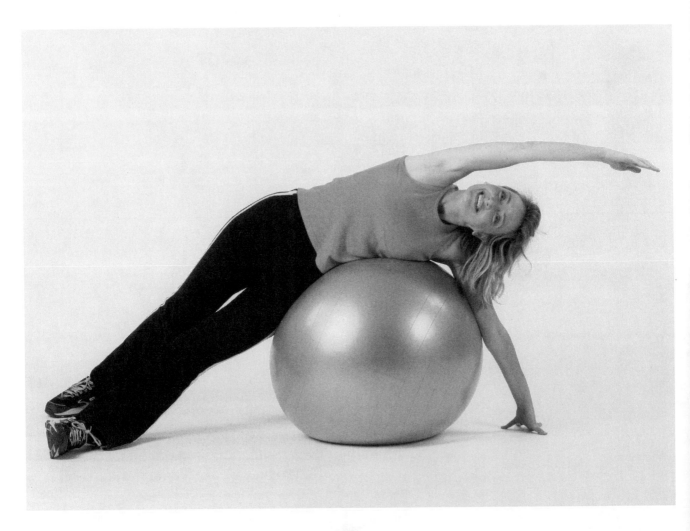

# Waist Stretch with Band

## TECHNIQUE & FORM

Sit on the floor with your feet far apart. Wrap the band around one of your feet and and hold it with the opposing hand. Rotate your body toward your foot and allow the band to assist in the stretch.

*Paul's Pro Tip*

Keep your back straight and rotate from the waist.

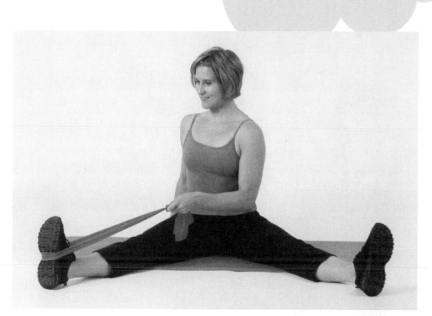

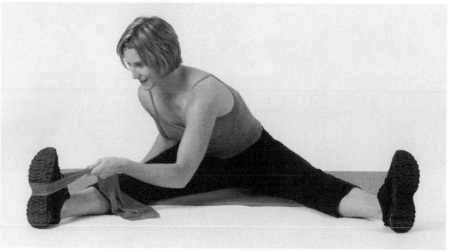

# Glute Stretch

**Paul's Pro Tip**

Increase the stretch by lowering your chest toward your knee.

## TECHNIQUE & FORM

Place the side of your bent knee on top of ball with the other leg extended behind you. Place both of your hands on the ball for added stability.

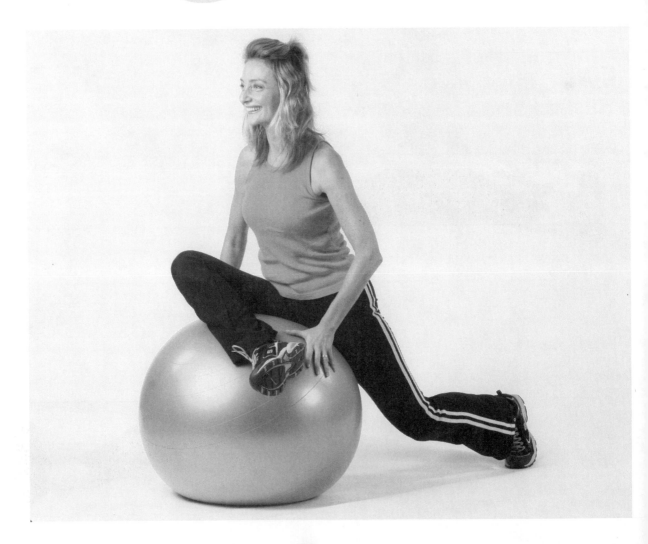

# Glute Stretch with Band

**Paul's Pro Tip**
Actively drawing your knee
toward your chest will allow a
deeper stretch.

**TECHNIQUE & FORM**
Lie on your back. Wrap the band across your ankle and draw your
knee towards the opposing shoulder.

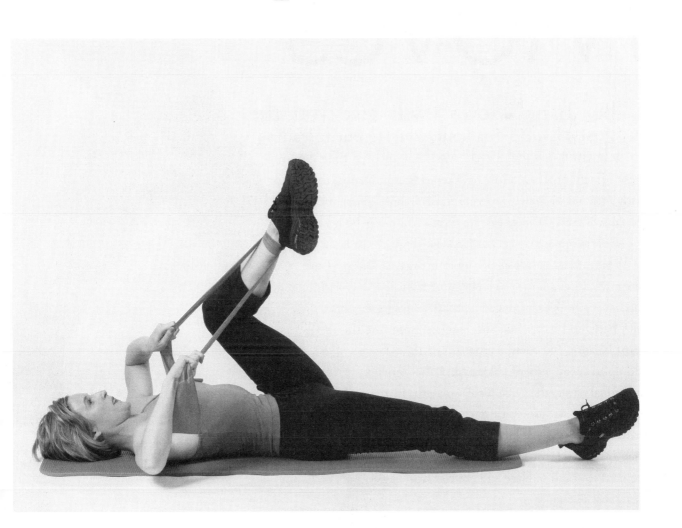

### Chapter 6

# Power Band Big Bang Moves

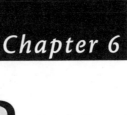

"Big Bang Moves" will give you the biggest results for your exercise buck, leading to a leaner, toned body with less of a time commitment. Each of the following exercises conditions the entire body (the upper, lower, and core musculature). These total body movements burn the most calories because the entire body exercises as a whole as opposed to isolating individual muscles by body part.

Which exercise consumes more energy, a Biceps Curl where the biceps muscle is isolated or a Biceps Curl with Alternating Backward Lunges? The latter engages the legs, butt, back, and biceps and also requires more core stability, balance, and coordination. All of these factors add up to spend a lot of calories and also develops functional strength. Functional strength is the strength that we use every day; in sports, at home, and on the job. After all, how often in your life outside of a gym have you been required to stand in place and exercise isolating just one muscle?

## The Exercises

# Trunk Upward Chop Lift

## (Weight Shift)

### TECHNIQUE & FORM

Stand with your feet shoulder width apart and your knees bent. Anchor the band at floor level and hold the band with both your hands. Shift your weight from one leg to the other. Rotate torso, keeping your hips fixed. Draw your arms up over the opposite shoulder, keeping your back straight and your chest high.

*This exercise can be performed with both the exercise band and tube.*

### Paul's Pro Tip

Begin the movement with your legs, not your hands. Keeping your arms straight, focus on your abdominals for the best workout.

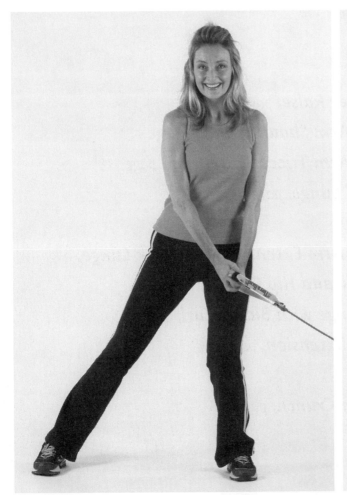
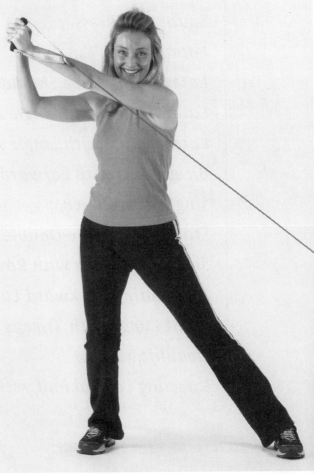

# Diagonal Ax Chop

*(Weight Shift)*

## TECHNIQUE & FORM

Stand with your feet shoulder width apart and your knees bent. Anchor the band at chest level and hold the band with both your hands. Shift your weight from one leg to another. Rotate torso, turning your shoulders with your arms parallel to the floor.

*This exercise can be performed with both the exercise band and tube.*

*Paul's Pro Tip*
Make sure to keep your head facing forward while rotating your trunk.

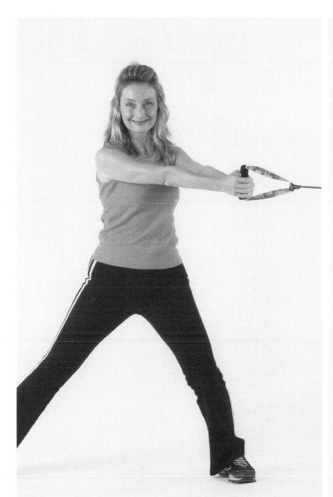
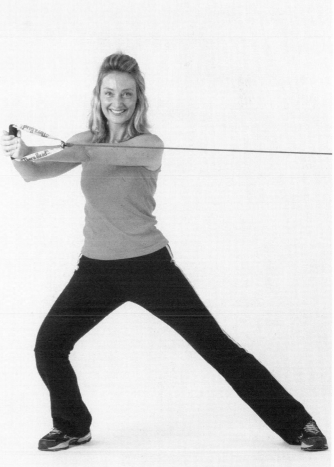

# Downward Ax Chop

### TECHNIQUE & FORM

Stand with both your feet shoulder width apart with your knee bent. Anchor the band overhead and hold the band with both of your hands. Shift your weight from one leg to the other. Rotate your torso, drawing the band to the opposing knee. Keep your hips fixed forward.

*This exercise can be performed with both the exercise band and tube.*

*Paul's Pro Tip*

Before beginning any ax chop movements, always draw your belly in tight.

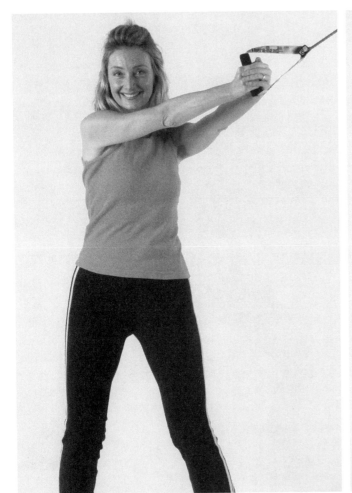
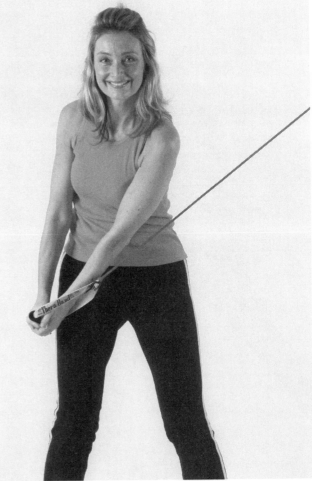

# Single Leg Backward Lunge with Row

## TECHNIQUE & FORM

Stand with your feet shoulder width apart. The band should be anchored at shoulder height. Hold the band in your hands with your arms extended in front of you. Lunge backward and simultaneously pull your arms back.

*This exercise can be performed with both the exercise band and tube.*

### Paul's Pro Tip

Changing the angle and the height of your arms from low to medium, to high changes which back muscles are exercised. See the next three variations for an example.

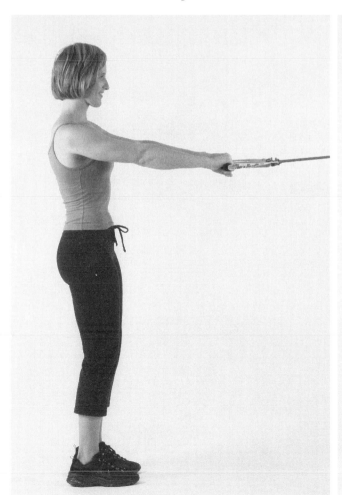
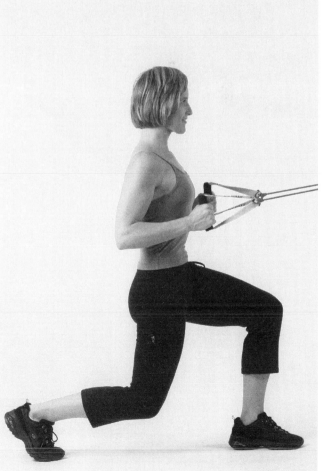

# Single Leg Front Lunge with Press

*This exercise can be performed with both the exercise band and tube.*

## TECHNIQUE & FORM
Stand with your feet shoulder width apart, your back to where the band is anchored at shoulder height. Holding the band in your arms, lunge forward with one leg and at the same time press and extend your arms in front of your chest. Return to the beginning position and repeat with the other leg leading.

*Paul's Pro Tip*
Keeping the shoulder blades back as you press the bands to the front will better engage the chest muscles.

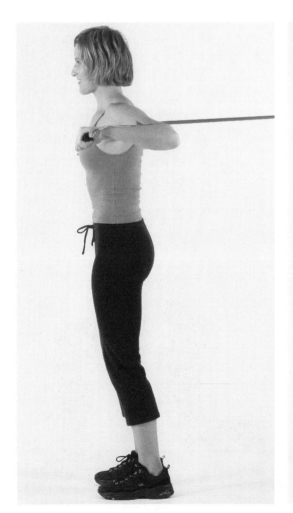
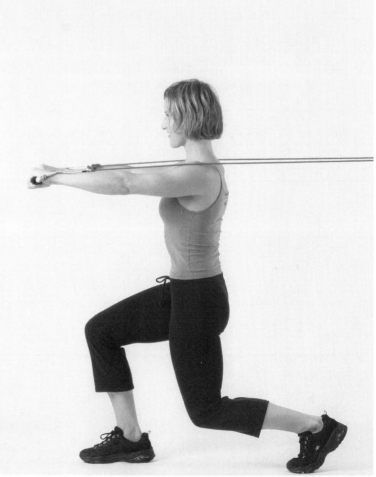

# Single Leg Backward Lunge with Upright Row

*This exercise can be performed with both the exercise band and tube.*

*Paul's Pro Tip*

Do not allow your shoulders to shrug upwards toward the ears during the rowing movement.

## TECHNIQUE & FORM

Stand with your feet shoulder width apart facing a band anchored at chest level. Lunge backward with one leg and row, keeping your elbows held high. Return to the starting position and repeat using the other leg.

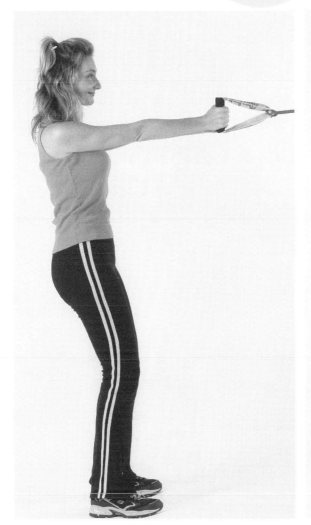

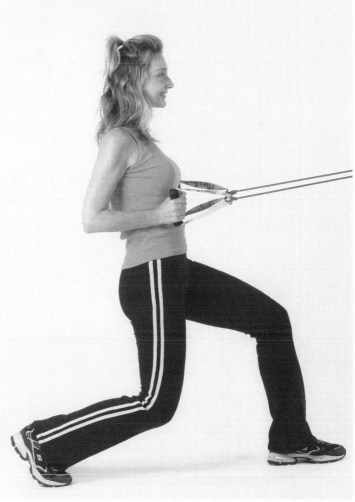

# Squat and Row

## TECHNIQUE & FORM
Anchor the band low on the floor and hold the band in your hands, extending your arms. Begin in a squat with your feet shoulder width or farther apart. When ready, simultaneously rise up from the squat and pull arms backward in a row.

*This exercise can be performed with both the exercise band and tube.*

*Paul's Pro Tip*
The backs of the thighs should be parallel to the floor when you are in the starting position.

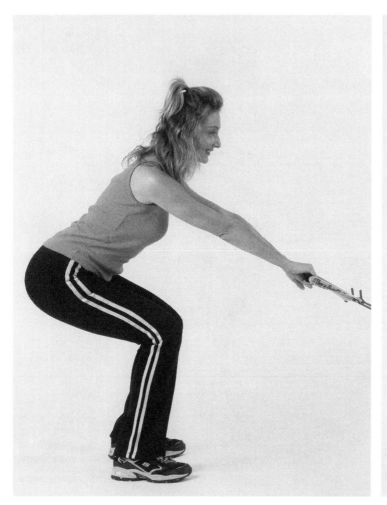
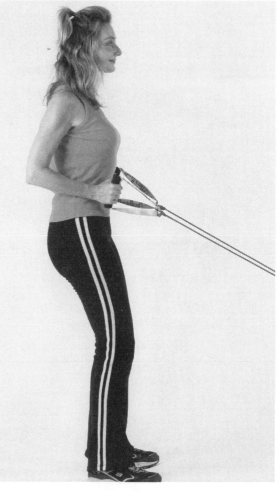

# Squat and Lateral Pull

## TECHNIQUE & FORM

Stand with your feet shoulder width apart, with the band anchored high. Hold the band in your hands and extend your arms overhead. Drop down into a squat and, at the same time, pull the band down toward you.

*This exercise can be performed with both the exercise band and tube.*

### Paul's Pro Tip

If you change how far apart you hold your arms, you will target different muscles in your back. The wider you hold your arms, the more difficult the exercise.

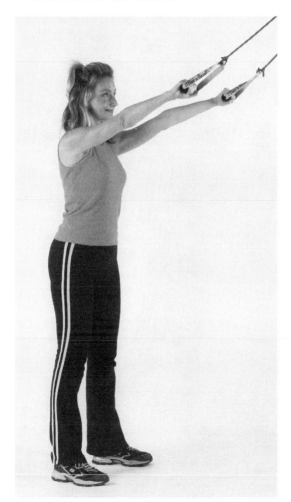

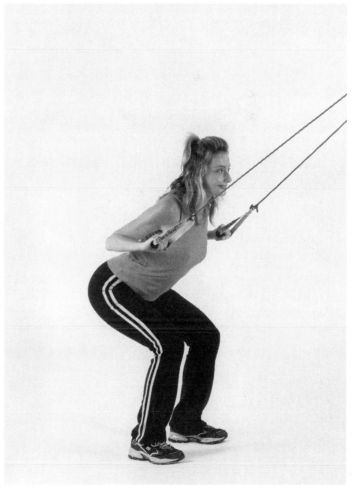

# Squat and Press

## TECHNIQUE & FORM
Begin this exercise in a squat with the band anchored low on the ground. Hold the band in your hands with your hands at shoulder height. As you rise up from the squat, press your hands overhead.

*This exercise can be performed with both the exercise band and tube.*

*Paul's Pro Tip*
Maintain the curvature in your lower back at all times with any squatting movement.

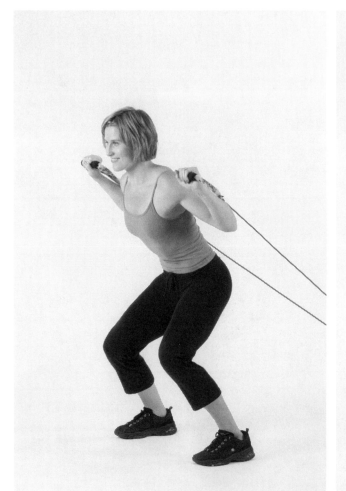
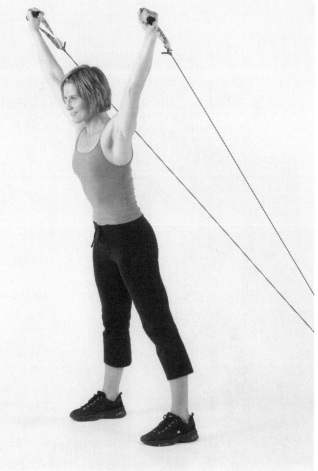

# Lateral Shift

*This exercise can be performed with both the exercise band and tube.*

### Paul's Pro Tip
Keep your chest held up high and avoid rolling your shoulder forward. Keep your focus on the outer and inner thighs.

## TECHNIQUE & FORM
Stand with your feet placed wide and the band anchored low and to the side. Hold the band in your hands with your arms held straight. Your starting position has the knees bent and your body weight shifted toward the band. Shift your weight so your body moves over the opposite knee.

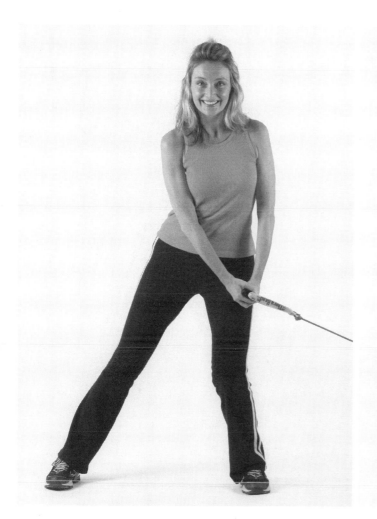
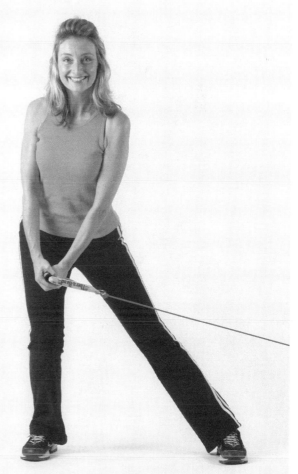

# Lateral Shift with Shoulder Raise

*This exercise can be performed with both the exercise band and tube.*

**Paul's Pro Tip**

Bend at the knees, not the waist. If flexibility is poor, try pointing your toes outward.

## TECHNIQUE & FORM

Stand with your feet placed wide and the band anchored low and to the side. Hold the band in your hands with your arms held straight. Start with the knees bent and the body weight shifted over the knee closest to the band. Now shift your weight so your body moves over the opposite knee. As your weight shifts, pull your elbows high.

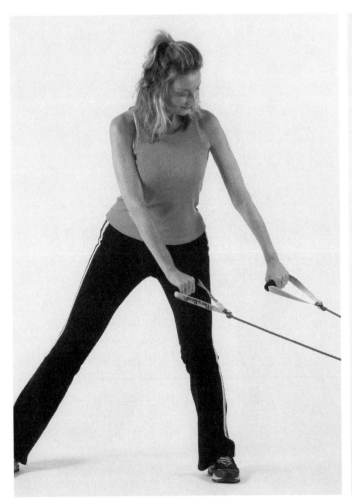
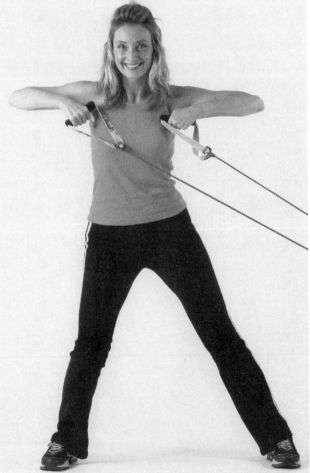

# Lateral Shift with Single Arm Shoulder Press

*This exercise can be performed with both the exercise band and tube.*

### Paul's Pro Tip

This exercise will target the sides of your waist. Be sure to keep your abdominals draw in tightly.

## TECHNIQUE & FORM

Stand with your feet placed wide and the band anchored low. Hold the band in one hand and at shoulder level. Beginning with your weight shifted towards the leg nearest the band, come up from the squat while pressing the band overhead and toward the opposite shoulder.

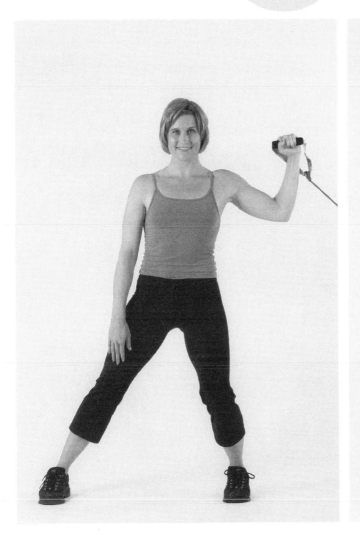
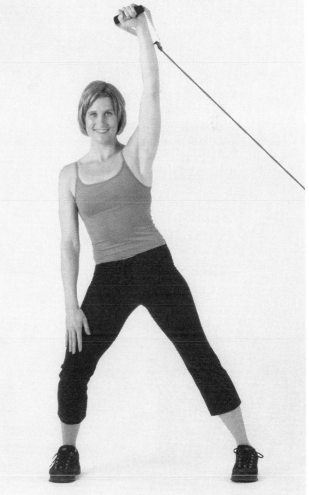

# Lateral Shift with Single Arm Triceps Extension

*This exercise can be performed with both the exercise band and tube.*

### Paul's Pro Tip

The pulling motion of the arm begins by pulling the elbow across the body, then ends by executing the triceps extension.

## TECHNIQUE & FORM

Stand with your feet placed wide and the band anchored high and to the side. Hold the band with the hand farthest away. The arm should come across your chest. Begin with your weight shifted toward the band and shift toward the opposite side, simultaneously pulling the band across your body and extending your arm out.

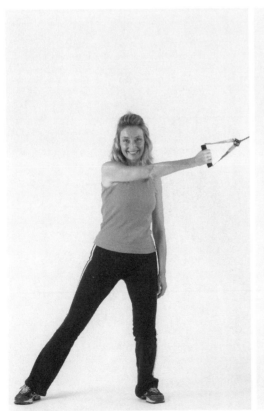 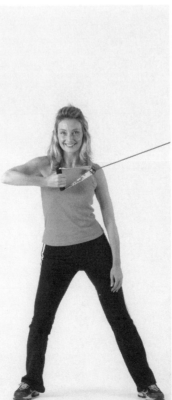 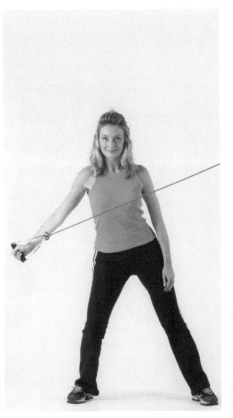

# Biceps Curl with Forward Lunge

*This exercise can be performed with both the exercise band and tube.*

### TECHNIQUE & FORM

Stand with your feet hip distance apart. The band is anchored low and from behind. Hold the band in your hands with your palms facing forward. Lunge forward with one leg and simultaneously perform a biceps curl. Return to the beginning position and alternate your legs.

*Paul's Pro Tip*

Keep your elbows close to your waist when performing the biceps curls.

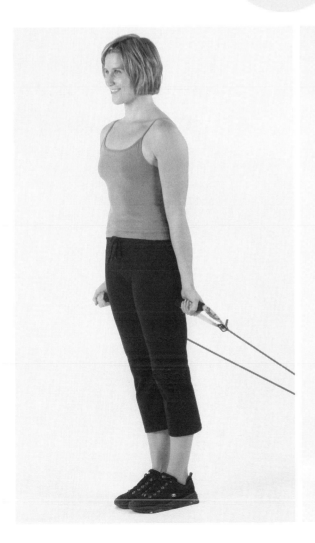

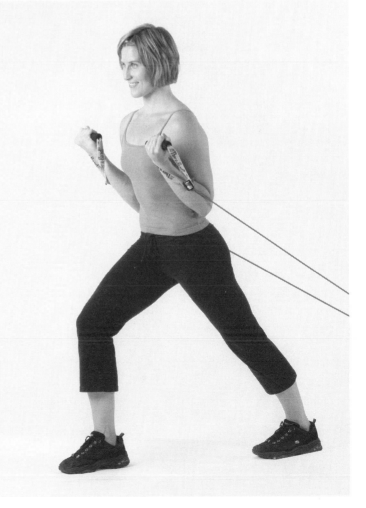

# Single Arm Punch

*This exercise can be performed with both the exercise band and tube.*

## TECHNIQUE & FORM
Stand with your feet spread wide, and anchor the band at shoulder height. Your side should face the band as you hold the band in one hand. Rotate away from band and drop into lunge as the arm holding the band extends into a punch.

*Paul's Pro Tip*
The leg and hips should initiate the movement, the punch following in a smooth motion.

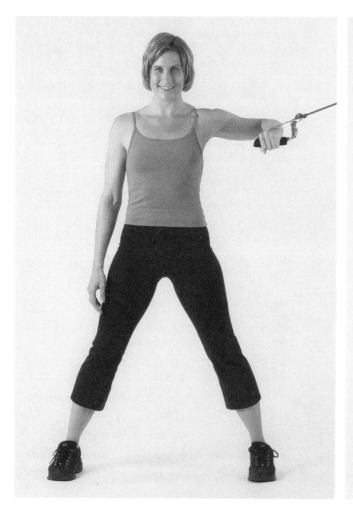

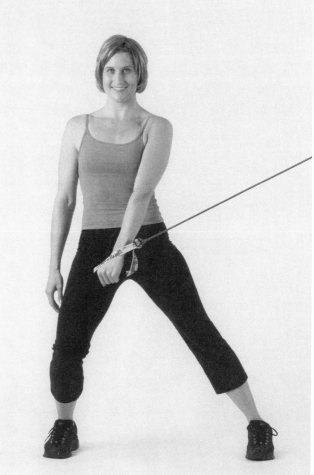

# Standing Reverse Double Arm Extension with Back Lunge

*This exercise can be performed with both the exercise band and tube.*

***Paul's Pro Tip***
Focus on bringing your shoulder blades together. Keep the shoulder down and away from your ears.

## TECHNIQUE & FORM

Stand with your feet hip distance apart. Anchor the band at chest level and hold the band with your arms extended in front of your chest. Keeping your arms straight, extend your arms backward while taking a backward lunge.

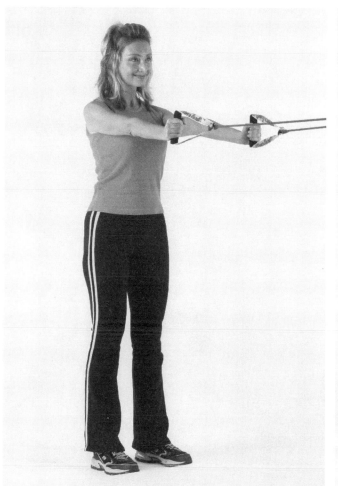
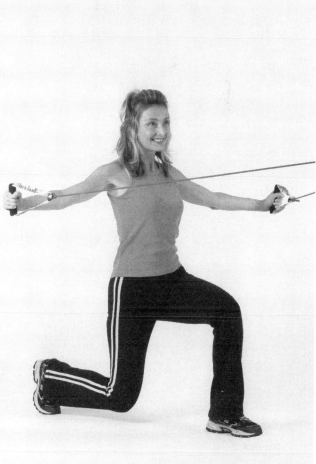

# Single Leg Lunge
# with Row and Hip Flexion

*This exercise can be performed with both the exercise band and tube.*

*Paul's Pro Tip*

Focus on keeping your belly drawn tight and avoid bending forward at the waist.

## TECHNIQUE & FORM

Begin in a lunge position with one arm extended. The band should be anchored overhead. Hold the band in one hand with your arm extended in front of your chest. Begin performing a single arm row, while drawing your back knee up to your chest. Return to starting position.

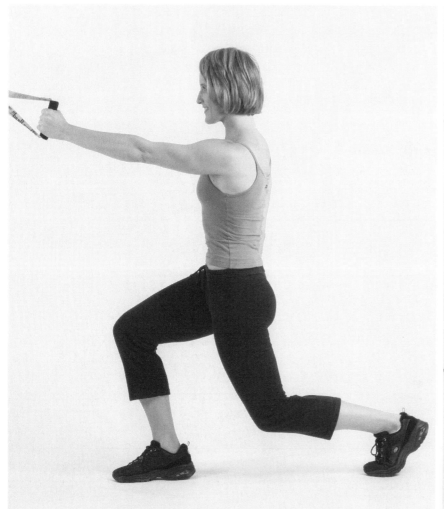
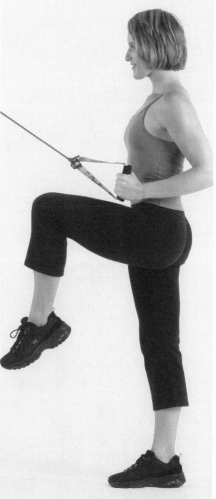

# Alternating Backward Lunge with Biceps Curl

*This exercise can be performed with both the exercise band and tube.*

### Paul's Pro Tip

Keep your elbow in a fixed position and your shoulders back. This will focus the exercise on your biceps.

## TECHNIQUE & FORM

Begin with your feet shoulder width apart and the band anchored at floor level. Hold the band with your hands held low. Take a backward lunge while performing a biceps curl. Return to the starting position and alternate your lunging leg.

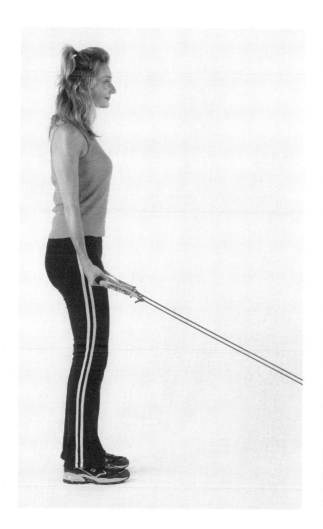
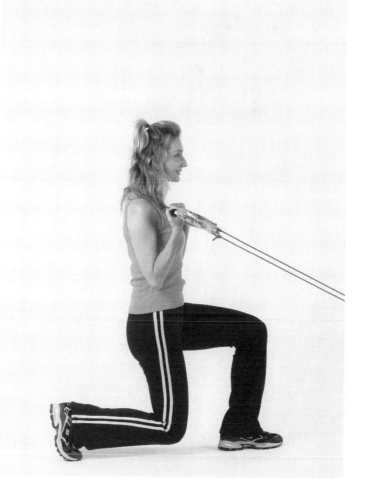

# Front Lunge
## with Triceps Extension

*This exercise can be performed with both the exercise band and tube.*

### Paul's Pro Tip
Keep your elbows facing forward with the backs of your arms held parallel to the floor.

### TECHNIQUE & FORM
Stand with your feet hip width apart, and the band anchored even with your head. Hold the band with both hands, arms bent at the elbow at 90 degrees, with the palms facing upward. Lunge forward and press the bands forward at the same time.

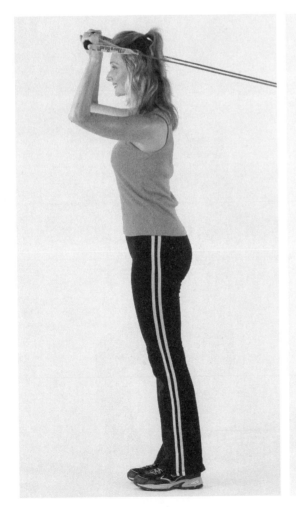

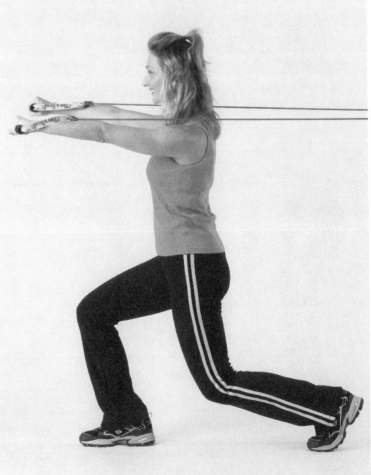

# Deadlift

*This exercise can be performed with both the exercise band and tube.*

## TECHNIQUE & FORM

Anchor the band at the floor. Stand with your feet shoulder width apart and your arms extended in front of your body. Bend forward at your waist and keep your knees slightly bent. Then straighten your legs and bring the torso to an upright position.

### Paul's Pro Tip

Keep your head in line with your spine. Draw your belly in tight and keep your shoulders back.

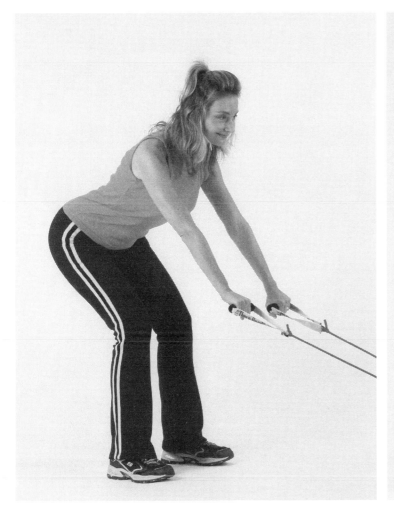
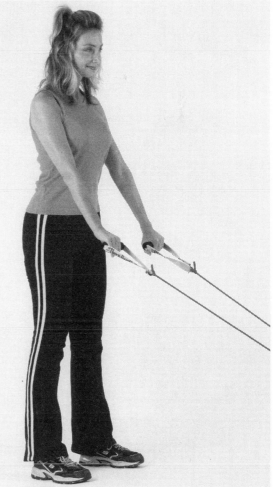

# Kneeling Lateral Pull with Crunch

*This exercise can be performed with both the exercise band and tube.*

### Paul's Pro Tip

If you allow the bands to stretch the arms high, this will also stretch the abdominal muscles and intensify the crunch.

## TECHNIQUE & FORM

Kneel on the floor. The band should be anchored overhead. Extend your arms above your head and grasp the band. Draw hands to the fronts of your shoulder, lowering your butt to your heels and bringing your chest toward your thigh.

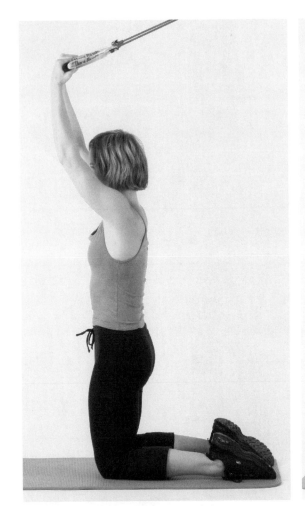

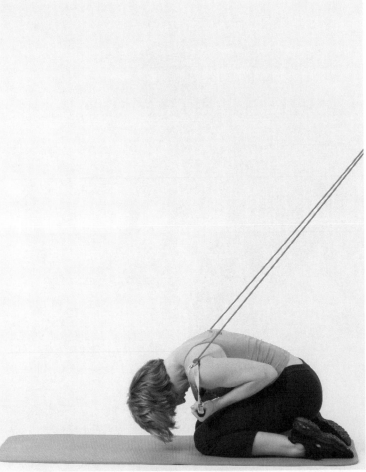

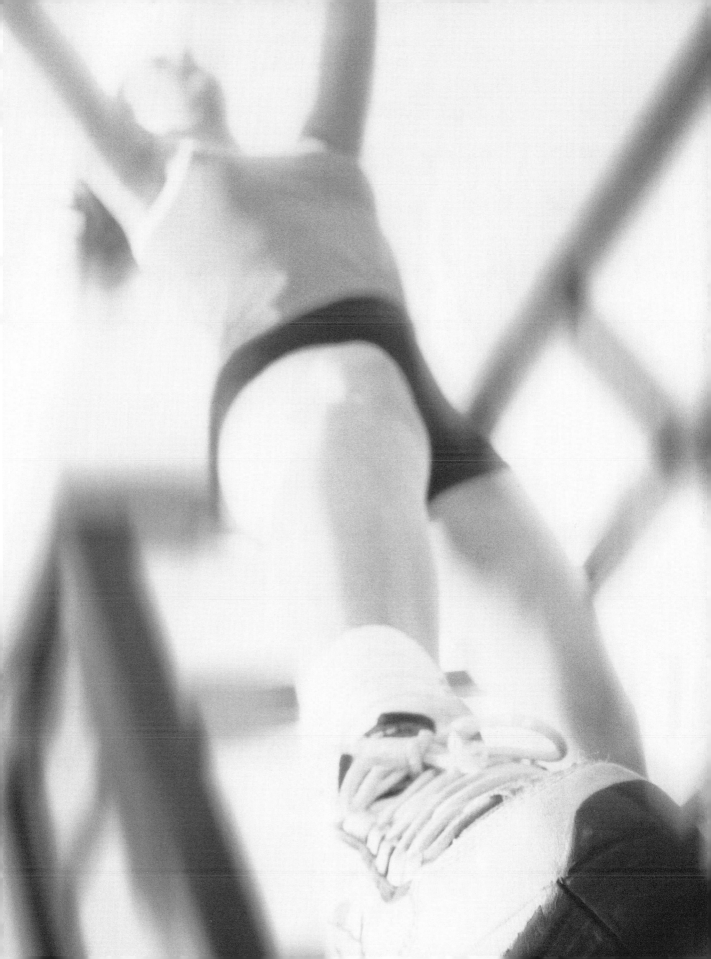

### Chapter 7

# The PowerBand Workouts

Following the PowerBand Workouts sequentially—starting with Stage I—is essential for developing a safe, effective, progressive, and successful training regimen. Here are some general points to keep in mind: No two individuals are alike. The number of reps and sets are general recommendations. The workouts should be challenging—not impossible. Never, ever, sacrifice form to complete a set. If you feel you need to repeat a week before moving on to the second, more challenging week, do so!

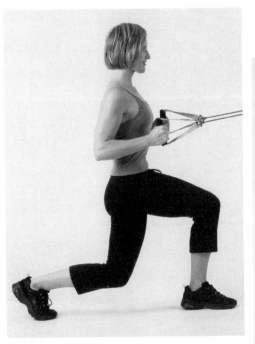
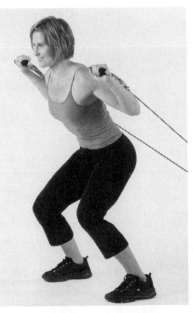
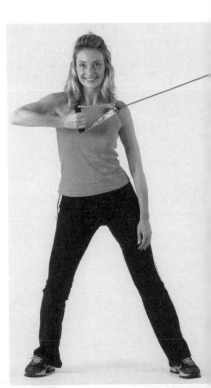

Remember to warm up every time before you exercise. An effective warm-up increases your heart rate and the blood flow to your muscles. Don't feel that you need to complete each exercise through the complete range of motion. Each exercise can—and should—be modified to fit your fitness level. Remember: Pain should never be part of your exercise program.

### Chapter 3
start on page 10

# Warm-Up

| | |
|---|---|
| Seated Ax Chop | 15X on each side |
| Seated Reverse Ax Chop | 15X on each side |
| Double Arm Punching | 30 seconds |
| Backward Lunge | 10X on each leg |
| Front Lunge | 10X on each leg |
| Lateral Lunge | 10X on each side |

Stretching post-workout is important every time you exercise. This is the time when you actually improve your flexibility—when your muscles are warmed up. Remember, if at any time you feel pain, stop. Don't feel as if you need to complete a stretch if your body says otherwise.

### Chapter 5
start on page 82

# Stretching

| | |
|---|---|
| Chest Stretch with Band | Hold 15-20 seconds |
| Triceps Stretch with Band | Hold 15-20 seconds |
| Quadriceps Stretch with Band | Hold 15-20 seconds |
| Hamstring Stretch with Band | Hold 15-20 seconds |
| Shoulder Stretch with Band | Hold 15-20 seconds |
| Biceps Stretch with Band | Hold 15-20 seconds |
| Upper Back Stretch with Band | Hold 15-20 seconds |
| Lower Back Stretch with Band | Hold 15-20 seconds |
| Waist Stretch with Band | Hold 15-20 seconds |
| Glute Stretch with Band | Hold 15-20 seconds |

# PowerBand Stage 1: Adaptation

This stage will introduce you to the feel of resistance training with the use of the band. Your task will be to keep the resistance at a manageable level and your focus on the target muscle. Once you feel you have a good sense of the movements required for each exercise, begin slowly adding additional resistance.

- Do three workouts per week for three weeks.
- Begin each workout with a 10-minute warm-up.
- Finish with 10 minutes of stretching.

| Week 1 | Arms | Week 2 |
|---|---|---|
| 2 x 15 Standing Biceps Curl | | 3 x 15 Standing Biceps Curl |
| 2 x 15 Standing Triceps Extention | | 3 x 15 Standing Triceps Extention |

| Week 1 | Shoulders | Week 2 |
|---|---|---|
| 1 x 15 Shoulder Lateral Raise | | 2 x 15 Shoulder Lateral Raise |
| 1 x 15 Shoulder Front Raise | | 2 x 15 Shoulder Front Raise |
| 1 x 15 Shoulder Rear Delt | | 2 x 15 Shoulder Rear Delt |

| Week 1 | Chest | Week 2 |
|---|---|---|
| 1 x 15 Chest Press with Band | | 2 x 15 Chest Press with Band |

| Week 1 | Back | Week 2 |
|---|---|---|
| 1 x 15 Middle-Back Standing Row | | 2 x 15 Middle-Back Standing Row |
| 1 x 15 Standing Lateral Pulldown | | 2 x 15 Standing Lateral Pulldown |

| Week 1 | **Legs** | Week 2 |
|--------|----------|--------|
| 1 x 15<br>Squat | | 2 x 15<br>Squat |

| | **Glutes** | |
|--------|----------|--------|
| 1 x 15<br>Four Ped Glutes (each leg) | | 2 x 15<br>Four Ped Glutes (each leg) |

| | **Hamstrings** | |
|--------|----------|--------|
| 1 x 15<br>Standing Hamstring | | 2 x 15<br>Standing Hamstring |

| | **Abs** | |
|--------|----------|--------|
| 2 x 20<br>Crunch | | 2 x 40<br>Crunch |
| 2 x 20<br>Seated Rotation<br>on Ball (each leg) | | 2 x 40<br>Seated Rotation<br>on Ball (each leg) |

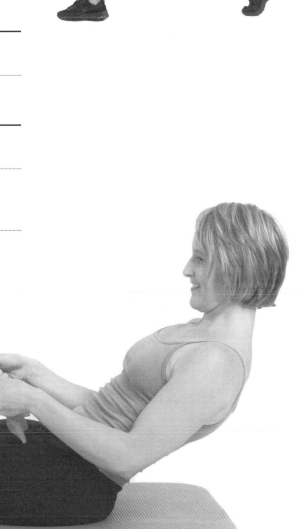

# PowerBand Stage 2: Strength

In Stage 2 you will overload your muscles with work. The workout is designed to target the same muscle with more than one exercise, and will hit the musculature at several different angles. This will help you develop fuller, stronger, and more defined muscles.

•Do three workouts per week for three weeks.

• Begin each workout with a 10-minute warm-up.

• Finish with 10 minutes of stretching.

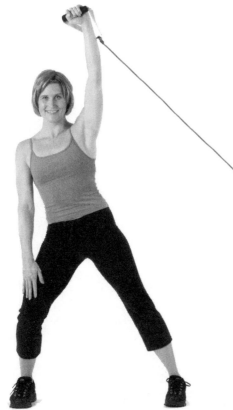

| Week 1 | Arms | Week 2 |
|---|---|---|
| 2 x 15 Standing Biceps Curl | | 3 x 15 Standing Biceps Curl |
| 2 x 15 Preacher Curl on Ball | | 3 x 15 Preacher Curl on Ball |
| 2 x 15 Standing Triceps Extension | | 3 x 15 Standing Triceps Extension |
| 2 x 15 Triceps Seated Extension on Ball | | 3 x 15 Triceps Seated Extension on Ball |

| | Shoulders | |
|---|---|---|
| x 15 Shoulder Lateral Raise | | 3 x 15 Shoulder Lateral Raise |
| x 15 Shoulder Front Raise | | 3 x 15 Shoulder Front Raise |
| 2 x 15 Shoulder Rear Delt | | 3 x 15 Shoulder Rear Delt |

| | Chest | |
|---|---|---|
| 2 x 15 Chest Press with Band | | 3 x 15 Chest Press with Band |
| 2 x 15 Chest Fly Bungee | | 3 x 15 Chest Fly Bungee |

| Week 1 | **Back** | Week 2 |
| --- | --- | --- |
| 2 x 15 Middle-Back Standing Row | | 3 x 15 Middle-Back Standing Row |
| 2 x 15 Upper Back Standing Row | | 3 x 15 Upper Back Standing Row |
| 2 x 15 Standing Lateral Pulldown | | 3 x 15 Standing Lateral Pulldown |

## Legs

| | |
| --- | --- |
| 2 x 15 Squat | 3 x 15 Squat |
| 2 x 15 Lunge | 3 x 15 Lunge |
| 2 x 15 Back Lunge | 3 x 15 Back Lunge |

## Glutes

| | |
| --- | --- |
| 2 x 15 Standing Glutes (each leg) | 3 x 15 Standing Glutes (each leg) |
| 2 x 15 Standing Abduction (each leg) | 3 x 15 Standing Abduction (each leg) |

## Hamstrings

| | |
| --- | --- |
| 2 x 15 Standing Hamstring | 3 x 15 Standing Hamstring |
| 2 x 15 Four Ped Hamstring | 3 x 15 Four Ped Hamstring |

## Abs

| | |
| --- | --- |
| 1 x 20 Crunch | 2 x 20 Crunch |
| 1 x 20 Lower Abs Crunch | 2 x 20 Lower Abs Crunch |
| 2 x 20 Seated Rotation on Ball (each side) | 2 x 20 Seated Rotation on Ball (each side) |

# PowerBand Stage 3: Endurance

Musculature endurance is your muscles' ability to work for pro-longed periods of time. This is what we're striving to achieve in Stage 3. Once you've reached this level, you may consider yourself an athlete-in-training. This is an excellent strength program for individuals preparing for athletic activities such as skiing, running, biking, hiking, or triathlons.

• Do three workouts per week for two weeks.

• Begin each workout with a 10-minute warm-up.

• Finish with 10 minutes of stretching.

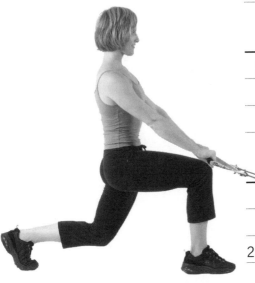

| Week 1 | Arms | Week 2 |
|--------|------|--------|
| 2 x 15 Standing Biceps Curl | | 3 x 15 Standing Biceps Curl |
| 2 x 15 Preacher Curl on Ball | | 3 x 15 Preacher Curl on Ball |
| 2 x 15 Standing Triceps Extension | | 3 x 15 Standing Triceps Extension |
| 2 x 15 Triceps Seated Extension on Ball | | 3 x 15 Triceps Seated Extension on Ball |
| 2 x 15 Tricep Extension Tabletop on Ball | | 3 x 15 Tricep Extension Tabletop on Ball |

| Week 1 | Shoulders | Week 2 |
|--------|-----------|--------|
| 2 x 15 Shoulder Lateral Raise | | 3 x 15 Shoulder Lateral Raise |
| 2 x 15 Shoulder Front Raise | | 3 x 15 Shoulder Front Raise |
| 2 x 15 Shoulder Rear Delt | | 3 x 15 Shoulder Rear Delt |

| Week 1 | Chest | Week 2 |
|--------|-------|--------|
| 2 x 15 Chest Press with Band | | 3 x 15 Chest Press with Band |
| 2 x 15 Chest Fly Bungee | | 3 x 15 Chest Fly Bungee |
| 2 x 15 Incline Chest Press on Ball | | 3 x 15 Incline Chest Press on Ball |

| Week 1 | Back | Week 2 |
|---|---|---|
| 2 x 15 Middle-Back Standing Row | | 3 x 15 Middle-Back Standing Row |
| 2 x 15 Upper Back Standing Row | | 3 x 15 Upper Back Standing Row |
| 2 x 15 Standing Lateral Pulldown | | 3 x 15 Standing Lateral Pulldown |
| 2 x 15 Standing Lateral Straight Arm Pulldown | | 3 x 15 Standing Lateral Straight Arm Pulldown |

## Legs

| Week 1 | Week 2 |
|---|---|
| 2 x 15 Squat | 3 x 15 Squat |
| 2 x 15 Lunge | 3 x 15 Lunge |
| 2 x 15 Back Lunge | 3 x 15 Back Lunge |

## Glutes

| Week 1 | Week 2 |
|---|---|
| 2 x 15 Standing Glutes (each leg) | 3 x 15 Standing Glutes (each leg) |
| 2 x 15 Standing Abduction (each leg) | 3 x 15 Standing Abduction (each leg) |
| 1 X 10 Steps Side Shuffle (both directions) | 2 x 10 Steps Side Shuffle (both directions) |

## Hamstrings

| Week 1 | Week 2 |
|---|---|
| 2 x 15 Standing Hamstring | 3 x 15 Standing Hamstring |
| 2 x 15 Four Ped Hamstring | 3 x 15 Four Ped Hamstring |
| 2 X 15 Supine Hamstring | 3 x 15 Supine Hamstring |

## Abs

| Week 1 | Week 2 |
|---|---|
| 1 x 20 Crunch | 2 x 20 Crunch |
| 1 x 20 Lower Abs Crunch | 2 x 20 Lower Abs Crunch |
| 2 x 20 Oblique Crunch on Ball (each side) | 2 x 20 Oblique Crunch on Ball (each side) |
| 1 x 20 Internal Oblique Crunch on Ball (each side) | 2 x 20 Internal Oblique Crunch on Ball (each side) |
| 1 x 20 Trunk Extension Sitting on Floor | 2 x 20 Trunk Extension Sitting on Floor |

# Big Bang "Body Attack" Workout

The PowerBand Big Bang Workouts are intensive body sculpting programs designed as supplements when the regular workout just isn't getting the results you want.

You want it all: strength, cardio, and endurance—but you don't want to spend all day at the gym. This, short, simple workout is the plan for you. It was designed for experienced exercisers with the band, so you may have to work up to be prepared for the intensity found in this routine.

## Beginner

1 x 10 Trunk Upward Chop Lift (Weight Shift)

1 x 10 Diagonal Ax Chop (Weight Shift)

1 x 10 Downward Ax Chop (each side)

1 x 10 Single Leg Front Lunge with Press

1 x 10 Single Leg Backward Lunge with Upright Row

1 x 10 Lateral Shift with Single Arm Shoulder Press

1 x 10 Alternating Backward Lunge with Biceps Curl

1 x 10 Front Lunge with Triceps Extension

2 x 10 Kneeling Lateral Pull with Crunch

## Intermediate

1 x 10 Trunk Upward Chop Lift (Weight Shift)

1 x 10 Diagonal Ax Chop (Weight Shift)

1 x 10 Downward Ax Chop (each side)

2 x 10 Single Leg Front Lunge with Press

2 x 10 Single Leg Backward Lunge with Upright Row

2 x 10 Lateral Shift with Single Arm Shoulder Press

2 x 10 Alternating Backward Lunge with Biceps Curl

2 x 10 Front Lunge with Triceps Extension

3 x 10 Kneeling Lateral Pull with Crunch

## *Advanced*

1 x 10 Trunk Upward Chop Lift (Weight Shift)

1 x 10 Diagonal Ax Chop (Weight Shift)

1 x 10 Downward Ax Chop (each side)

3 x 10 Single Leg Front Lunge with Press

3 x 10 Single Leg Backward Lunge with Upright Row

3 x 10 Lateral Shift with Single Arm Shoulder Press

3 x 10 Alternating Backward Lunge with Biceps Curl

3 x 10 Front Lunge with Triceps Extension

3 x 10 Kneeling Lateral Pull with Crunch

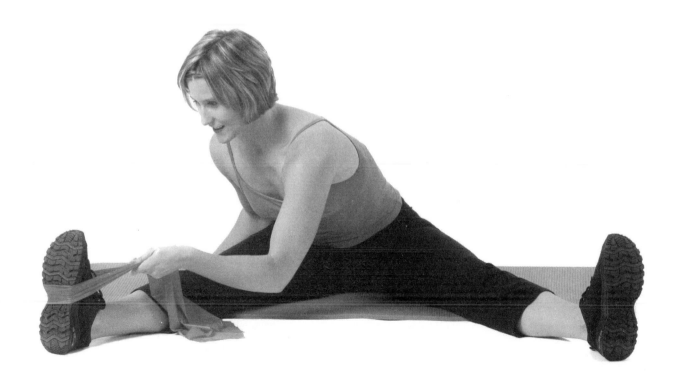

# Big Bang "Good Morning" Workout

The "Good Morning" Workout is an excellent energy booster. Not only is it great in the mornings, but it's great for avoiding those afternoon slumps. You can also use this routine as a warm-up for certain sports activities, like golf or tennis.

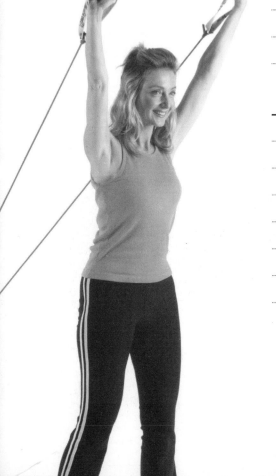

## Beginner

1 x 10 Trunk Upward Chop Lift (Weight Shift)

1 x 10 Diagonal Ax Chop (Weight Shift)

1 x 10 Downward Ax Chop (each side)

2 x 10 Squat and Row

2 x 10 Squat and Press

2 x 10 Deadlift

2 x 10 Kneeling Lateral Pull with Crunch

## Advanced

1 x 10 Trunk Upward Chop Lift (Weight Shift)

1 x 10 Diagonal Ax Chop (Weight Shift)

1 x 10 Downward Ax Chop (each side)

3 x 10 Squat and Row

3 x 10 Squat and Press

3 x 10 Deadlift

3 x 10 Kneeling Lateral Pull with Crunch